The
Cellulite-Free
Body

The Cellulite-Free Body

LARRY H. MELAMERSON

G. P. PUTNAM'S SONS   NEW YORK

Designed by Bernard Schleifer

Library of Congress Cataloging in Publication Data

Melamerson, Larry H   1953–
  The cellulite free body.

  Bibliography: p.
  1. Reducing exercises.   2. Exercise for
women.   I. Title.
RA781.6.M441   1981   613′.1   80-22677
ISBN 0-399-12527-2

Special thanks to those who helped me along the way:

Jane Rodrigues	Roy Scheider
Mart Crowley	Robert Carreiro
James Gabal	Ivo Lupis
Ron Najman	Walter Rozhen
Dean Pitchford	Howard Ronder
Swami Bua Ji Maharaj M.H.Y.	

Illustrations designed and drawn by Jeri Montalvo

Photos taken by Jeannette Montgomery

Exercises modeled by Joyce Forst, teacher of Physical Education and Choreography, New York City Public School System

Contents

Foreword

LARRY MELAMERSON CHANGED MY LIFE.

That is why I recommend this book to you, why I believe it will help you if you—like most women—have a cellulite problem. Just as I spend my life in fashion caring about beauty and design, Larry has devoted his life to physical fitness and health.

In April 1978, I had finished my fall collection and was utterly exhausted. Fall is the biggest and most important of the four women's collections I do each year. It involves months of work: designing; choosing fabrics, colors, buttons and trims; fitting each of the outfits and pieces several times on a model. Then there is the show: we work around the clock, making certain that everything is finished, that each outfit suits the model who will wear it on the runway—and that the music, the lighting, and the line-up are perfect.

The pressure doesn't end after the show. Then I deal with the press: the interviews, photography sessions, and the problems that inevitably arise, as when two fashion magazines demand exclusive rights to photograph the very same outfit.

I was so drained after the fall show in 1978 that I went to a spa in Mexico that stresses healthy living—simple food, regular exercise and early nights.

Back in New York, I didn't want to lose that feeling, so I went to Nicholas Kounovsky's Gym to ask about their program. Fortunately for me, Larry was there and he became my instructor.

At first I worked with him an hour a day, three days a week. As I grew stronger, I did an hour and a half, five days a week, of what became a combination of weightlifting, yoga and gymnastics. Eventually I built a gym next to my office, and Larry now coaches me there daily.

The routine he developed for me changed not just my body, but also my whole approach to life.

There's no doubt about my looking better. My weight is on my chest, shoulders, arms and legs—instead of on my stomach. My skin, which is naturally oily, is much clearer.

But the most important change that occurs when I exercise happens inside my head. It's almost like meditation. When I finish, my mind is much clearer. I am more relaxed and I am able to do more things. And if I go into the gym with a tension headache, it disappears after 10 or 15 minutes.

I look forward to exercising for the rest of my life. It has become automatic with me—I exercise just as I brush my teeth and take a shower.

What's more, I hope exercise will become automatic for my 14-year-old daughter Marci. Larry has worked out a routine to help her with specific problems. Like most teenagers, she needs to build confidence in herself. It took Larry a while to get her to believe she could do certain exercises. But now she is at the point where she trusts herself and will take a chance. As a result Marci is much better at sports—and delighted with her progress.

Larry has worked out the exercises for this book just as thoroughly as he worked out the routines for Marci and me. These exercises will help you rid yourself of ugly cellulite on your hips, thighs and buttocks.

The routine takes only 10 minutes a day—just a little more than an hour a week—to firm your muscles, break up fatty tissues and bring back your young, smooth-looking skin. There is no real excuse not to do them. Even if you spend your life in jeans, you'll look a lot better with slimmer thighs and a tighter backside.

People often ask me why I don't make clothes for women as large as size 14. I always have the same answer: I make clothes in sizes 2 to 12 because I believe a woman who cares about fashion also cares about her body. She keeps it slim and she keeps it in shape.

With Larry's exercises, you can too.

—CALVIN KLEIN

*The
Cellulite-Free
Body*

Introduction

CELLULITE IS AN IMPORTANT SUBJECT for women, and one that I take very seriously. Over the past seven years, I have been teaching exercise classes at the finest, most prestigious fitness studios in America: Rena of Chicago, Alex and Walter of Beverly Hills, Robert Carreiro of West Hollywood. I am presently associated with the most renowned studio in the world—Kounovsky Physical Fitness Center of Mid-Manhattan. The studios have been my laboratories, since they have presented me with the opportunity to study the effects of cellulite firsthand. The Bibliography in the back of this book represents three years of research in the libraries and bookstores of Northwestern, UCLA, Columbia, and New York universities.

In my years of teaching various women's exercise classes, the same question always arises: "How can I get rid of this dimpled, uneven fat around my hips, buttocks, and thighs?" In the beginning of my teaching days, I didn't really have a very good reply. When I was a physical-education student in college, the word *cellulite* was never mentioned. There weren't any books in English on the subject until Nicole Ronsard's *Cellulite,* which was an excellent source, except that it left a few questions unanswered. Therefore, I felt another book was needed to explain why some women develop cellulite while others don't, why a woman can be physically fit and still have cellulite, why skinny women develop cellulite even though they don't eat very much, and why exercise and diet aren't always as effective as they should be. *The Cellulite-Free Body* answers these questions and more, by explaining what most of you do wrong when you exercise and diet.

The Cellulite-Free Body describes a specially designed program that focuses on the trouble areas where cellulite may form. The program requires no special equipment or previous knowledge. All you need is a desire to look and feel good. The program is designed to break up fatty tissues, establish firm muscles, and bring back the young, smooth-looking skin you used to have before cellulite appeared. To accomplish this, I have created the cellulite-free-body exercise routine, which consists of thirty-four exercises, each designed to work a different area of the hips, buttocks, and thighs. The routine is divided into three programs: beginner, intermediate, and advanced. Regardless of your level of fitness, you can do it.

The cellulite-free-body exercise and diet routines have been proven on the flabbiest bottoms, the widest saddlebag hips, and the softest cottage cheese thighs that I could find. Every woman who stayed on the diet and exercised at least *one hour a week* without deviating from proper form lost all of her cellulite within ninety days. When they started, these women were no more than twenty pounds over their normal weight in accordance with their age and height.

The routines are extremely concentrated, designed to yield the utmost results in the shortest amount of time, giving you the cellulite-free body you always wanted but couldn't have before, taking only one hour a week, or ten minutes a day, to work!

What Is Cellulite and When Does It Form?

CELLULITE IS THE FRENCH NAME given to fat that changes in appearance. Cellulite and fat are essentially the same matter, but they take on different forms. Fat is smooth and clean and adds contour to a woman's body, while cellulite is organized in clumps of different gelatinous patterns ranging from a simple dimple to a cluster. Cellulite is found in places where the local flow of circulation has become stagnant, usually caused by poor posture, postural fault, and lack of proper exercise. Cellulite is a more difficult problem to solve than normal-looking fat, for it develops mostly around the hips, buttocks, and thighs, where general exercise and diet have little effect. I have designed the program described in *The Cellulite-Free Body* to help you with one of the most troublesome beauty problems in existence today!

You can first develop cellulite after the age of puberty, when the female hormone estrogen is produced by the ovaries. Estrogen creates the secondary sex characteristics that cause you to change from an adolescent into a woman, giving you the physical ability to bear children. Estrogen brings about the following changes in your body: the presence of a uniform layer of subcutaneous fat over the body; the tendency for adipose tissue (fat) to concentrate in the hips, buttocks, and thighs; a broader pelvis that increases your

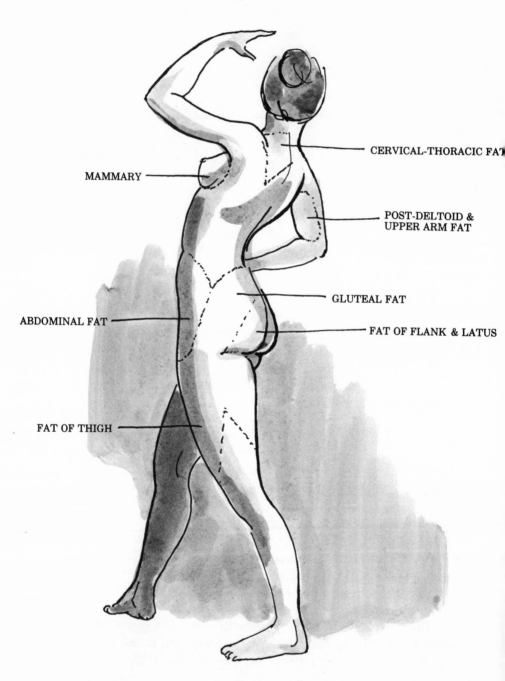

CERVICAL-THORACIC FAT

MAMMARY

POST-DELTOID &
UPPER ARM FAT

GLUTEAL FAT

ABDOMINAL FAT

FAT OF FLANK & LATUS

FAT OF THIGH

Fat distribution on the female figure.

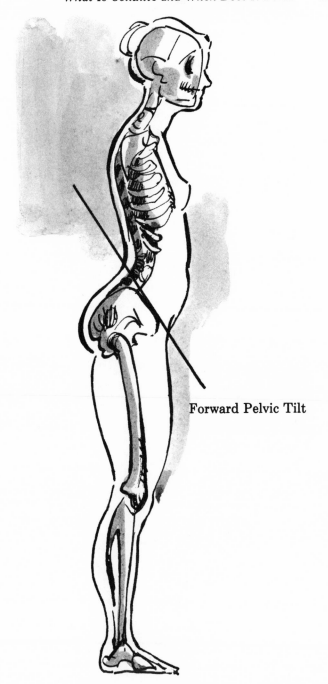

Forward Pelvic Tilt

Lordosis.

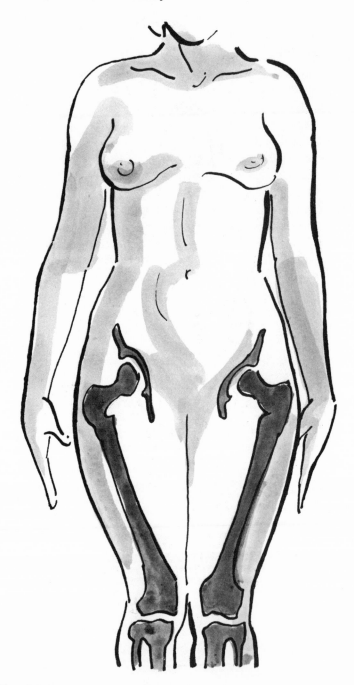

Knock-knee.

chances for lordosis (spinal and pelvic deviation); and a greater curvature of the thighbones that increases your chances for knock-knee (leg and knee deviation). These two postural faults, lordosis and knock-knee, combined with abundance of adipose tissue and subcutaneous fat, make the perfect formula for developing cellulite.

Cellulite is fat that deviates from the accepted form, which differs from normal-looking fat only in shape and texture. Cellulite develops around the hip joint, where the head of the thighbone connects into the pelvis. It mostly concentrates itself near the trochanter major (the bony projection below the neck of the thighbone), and can also be found in other areas of your body, depending on the following factors:

1. The efficiency of your local circulation systems (cardiovascular and lymphatic)
2. The degree of thickness between the subcutaneous adipose tissue (fat) layers and the connective tissue (fascia and muscle) layers
3. The degree that estrogen and other female hormones play in water retention, fat accumulation, and fat formation
4. The degree and kind of postural fault your body exhibits.

All these factors are determined by your secondary sex characteristics and by how well you take care of yourself in your posture, diet, and exercise practices.

Why Cellulite Forms: Postural Fault

THE HUMAN CIRCULATORY SYSTEM is a closed circuit, an ocean of fluid flowing in a circle of vessels. The circle is shaped by posture, and the fluid that flows within the circle is affected by posture. For example, if you were to pour cooking grease down the kitchen sink, it would turn from a liquid state into a solid state, hardening in the drain and clogging the pipe. The shape of the drainpipe is a determining factor, because it is not straight but u-shaped, which causes the grease to collect and eventually clog the pipe. The shape of the pipe influences the flow and drainage of materials. When it gets clogged, drain cleaners are needed to melt and loosen the grease. The human body is an intricate and complex mechanism, however, and swallowing a solvent to dissolve cellulite is not the answer—particularly since the inherent cause is structural and not functional.

Postural fault causes fat to be altered in appearance to another form, known as cellulite fat. When a woman is structurally balanced, centered with the gravitational forces which act upon her body, then her chances for developing cellulite are not very strong, even though she doesn't follow a good exercise or diet program. This is why some women don't have to diet and exercise as much as others. The drainpipe image illustrates how cellulite can form when there is a lack of

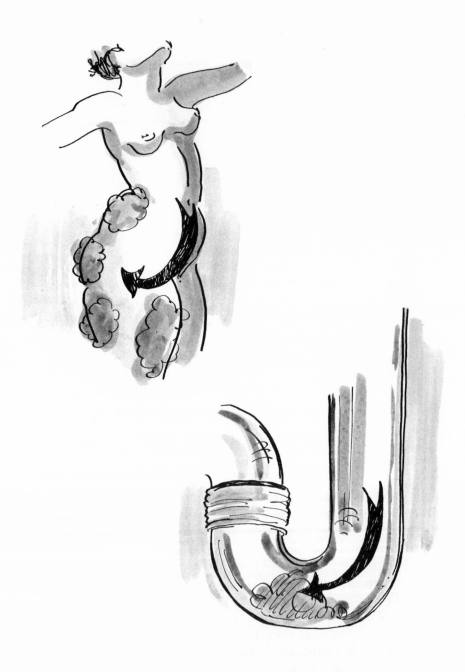

Drainpipe concept.

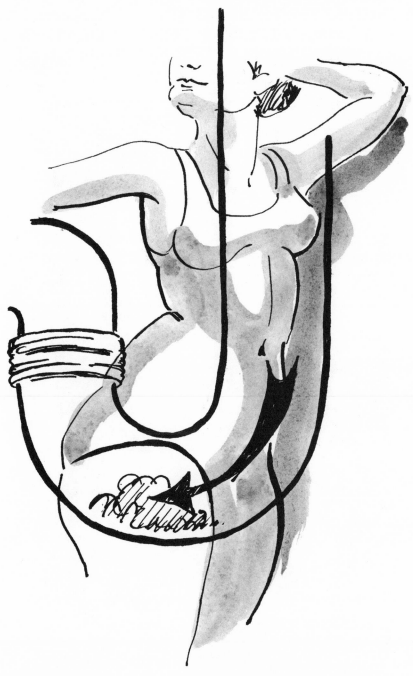

Drainpipe concept.

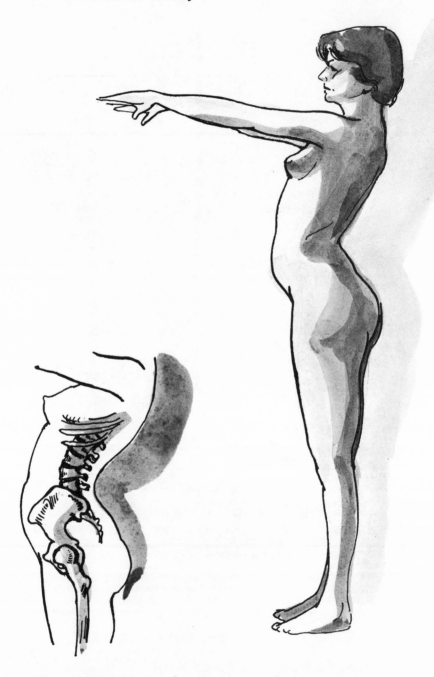

Postural fault/Lordosis.

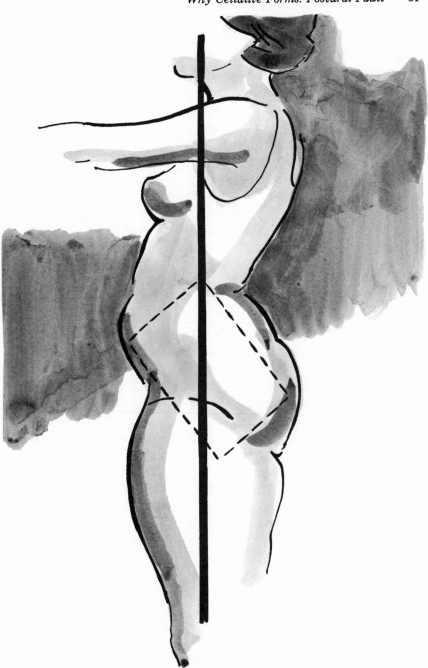

Forward pelvic tilt/Lordosis.

adequate circulation in a certain area caused by postural fault.

Every woman who has cellulite exhibits some form of *lordosis* (postural fault), an excessive forward curvature of the lower back and the top of the pelvis is tilted forward. Lordosis is caused by an increase in the angle (obliquity) of the sacrum. The sacrum is a bone that forms the base of the vertebral column, and acts as a bridge between the two halves of the pelvis. The lumbar curve compensates for the obliquity (tilt) of the upper end of the sacrum (which always slants downward and forward). The sacrum is slightly more oblique in women than in men, and consequently the lumbar curve is slightly greater in women than in men. A slight lordosis does not necessarily cause cellulite unless it is combined with poor diet, bad posture, and a lack of proper exercise.

Lordosis does add beauty and shape to a woman's body, for it creates the female curve. The *Playboy*-model type usually exhibits more than just a slight lordosis with her long torso, hyperextended lower back, small waist, extended hips, protruding buttocks, and a forward pelvic tilt, all of which adds up to that special curve men find attractive; but functionally, lordosis becomes a disadvantage as one of the main causes of cellulite.

With lordosis, the spine and pelvis deviate from the center line, making the back, hips, buttocks, and leg muscles tight and the stomach muscles weak. This causes the lower back and frontal thighs to take on most of the strain in

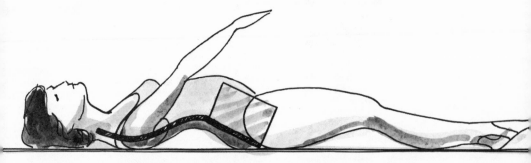

Lumbar-flattening (pushing the lower back and pelvis downward).

exercise, while the buttocks, hips, and outer thighs receive very little exercise. The cellulite-free-body exercise routine is specially designed to keep you from using your frontal-thigh and lower-back muscles by teaching you to use a medial and inward leg rotation technique, which will be discussed in Chapter 6. In addition, lumbar-flattening and pelvic-tucking techniques are mentioned later in this chapter.

Lordosis shifts the body's center of gravity in such a way that the gravitational center line falls behind the ideally aligned erect posture, which also causes the weight distribution (fat accumulation) to fall behind the center line. That means that most of your excess weight collects in the hips, buttocks, and outer thighs, in the form of cellulite. The degree of lordosis you exhibit and how you compensate for it will determine how the cellulite will take shape and form in your body.

In extreme cases of lordosis, there can be as much as four inches of vertical space between the floor and the highest point in the lumbar curve while a person is lying down on a flat surface in a supine position (on the back). Such excessive curvature elongates and stretches the *abdominals* (stomach muscles) and tightens the *iliopsoas* (hip and thigh flexors), *hamstrings* (hip and leg extensors), and *gluteals* (hip and buttock extensor and rotator muscles), which can cause lower-back pain and femoral and sciatic-nerve pains down the hips, buttocks, and legs.

If you have a lower-back problem, then you should check

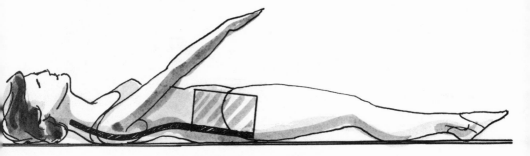

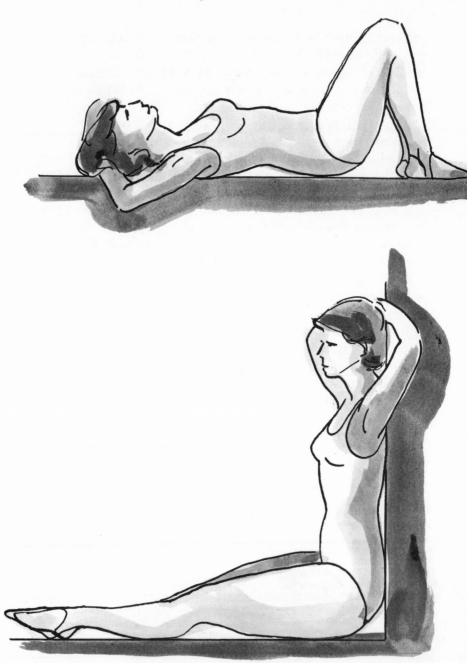

Lumbar-flattening and pelvic-tucking techniques.

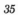

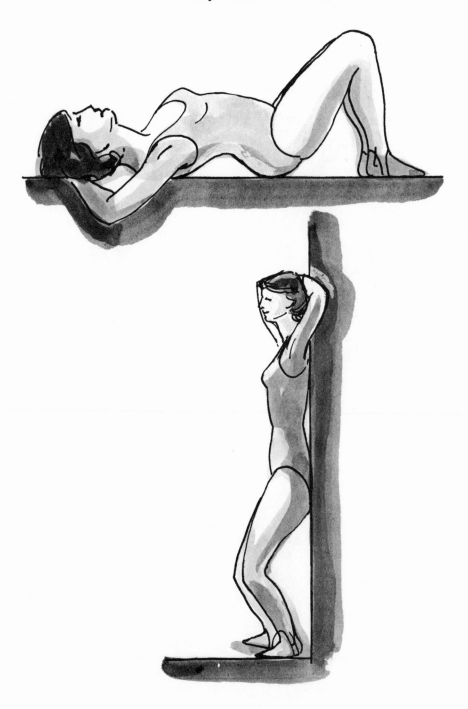

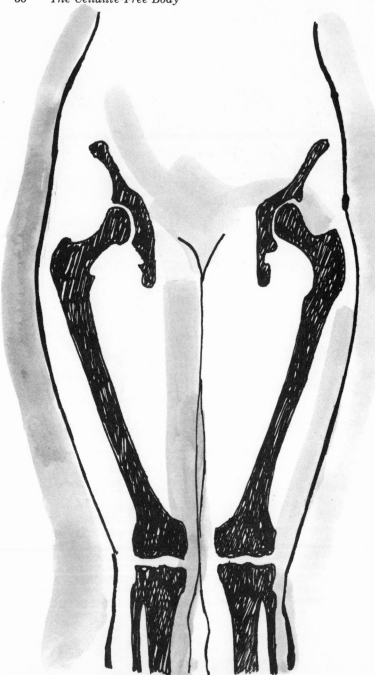

Knock-knee (femur obliquity).

with your doctor before starting the cellulite-free-body exercise routine, even though this program is specially designed for lower-back sufferers. It is better to be safe than sorry when it comes to your spine.

Lumbar flattening (backward pelvic tilting) is a basic technique, which is used to neutralize lordosis during exercise. By flattening out your lower back when you are lying on the floor, and by tucking your pelvis (hips) under when you are in a standing position, you can better align and center yourself. This technique helps improve posture and keeps lordosis under control.

Every woman who has an extreme case of cellulite also exhibits a postural fault called "knock-knee," a condition in which the legs bend inward, causing the knees to touch while the feet are apart. There are many infants who go through a period of knock-knee and lordosis, and most grow out of it by the age of four to seven years, depending on their structural maturity. Those who never correct the knock-knee and lordosis conditions are more likely to develop cellulite, unless a good diet, exercise, posture, and alignment program is followed.

How Cellulite Forms:
Sedentary Living

MODERN SOCIETY HAS CREATED an ideal environment for women to develop cellulite. Today most women work and live under sedentary and stressful conditions. Occupationally, women spend most of their days sitting or standing in one area behind a counter or desk. Sitting on furniture all day tightens, stiffens, and shortens the hips, buttocks, thighs, and lower leg muscles. Standing in one place all day also tightens and stiffens the body and causes poor circulation. Varicose veins (bulging and swollen veins in the legs) are an example of what years of standing in one place can do.

The body is a collection of various muscle groups, each one having its own particular role in the movement of the body. If a certain muscle group is not used, it will waste away (atrophy) and lose tone, and the unused area will turn to fat. The hips, buttocks, thighs, and lower leg muscles evolved from a need to move the body up from the ground, creating six basic body movements: kicking, sitting, climbing, crawling, squatting, and standing up. These movements are so basic that infants must learn them sequentially before they can walk properly. The body needs exercise for these muscle groups if it is to maintain its youth, mobility, and shape. The location of these muscles just happens to be where cellulite forms. Women in today's society rarely climb, crawl, squat, or

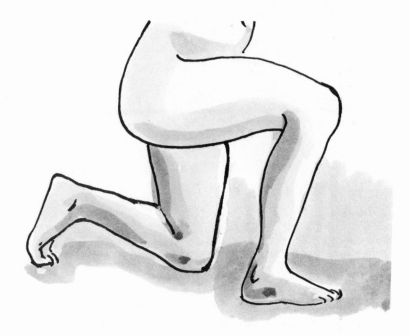

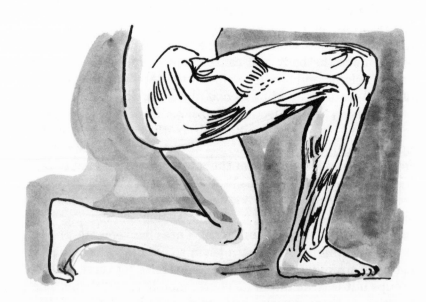

Muscles of the hips, buttocks, and legs.

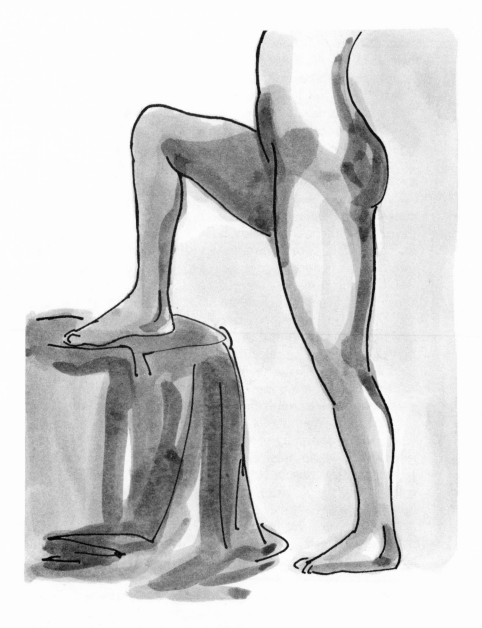

Side view of the hips, buttocks, and legs.

stand up from the ground. Since the muscles which cause these movements are not used as they were meant to be, they become flabby and unattractive.

Now I cannot ask you to climb, crawl, squat, or stand up from the ground, because it is not customary for adults to behave that way, and if you did, people would think you were acting childish, drunk, or even crazy and belong behind locked doors! Yet I can suggest that you practice the cellulite-free-body exercise routine, because it is the most sensible way to exercise your hips, buttocks, and thighs.

There are other exercises. The one best known to most people is walking, but one hour a week, or for that matter even an hour every day, will not get rid of your cellulite, because simply walking, swimming, or playing tennis are not concentrated enough. These forms of exercise don't work every hip, buttock, or thigh muscle in the body sufficiently, and they don't work the muscles through the *full range of motion* that is necessary to be totally effective against cellulite. The full-range-of-motion principle is based on working the muscle from its attachment of *origin* (the end of the muscle that attaches to a fixed point) to its attachment of *insertion* (the other end of the muscle that is attached to a movable point). The cellulite-free-body exercise routine does work all the muscles of the hips, buttocks, and thighs through a full range of motion in a concentrated manner. The routine gives the whole muscle of each muscle group a workout from its insertion. Walking, swimming, or tennis, for example, work mostly the belly of the muscles, and cellulite develops around the whole muscle, not just the belly. Exercise must put the entire muscle through a full range of motion to be fully effective in working the areas where cellulite can develop.

The proof of my findings can be found on many female athletes engaged in high-school, college, or professional sports, who have not exercised through a full range of motion. I have worked with some of these athletes who suffer from cellulite, and every one of them had some form of lordosis and a moderate to extreme case of knock-knee. But with my program, every one of them was cellulite-free within thirty days, because they were all able to start with the advanced exercises and high numbers of repetitions, which is not recommended unless you are in excellent physical condition. At the same time, they didn't have a serious weight problem to deal with, which is a very important factor in achieving quick results.

4

Why Cellulite Forms Even Though You Exercise

PEOPLE AREN'T REALLY AWARE of the way they move their bodies and the improper habits they have developed. In general, they choose the easiest way to do something if they think they are doing it right. However, what is physically right for one person may not be right for another. Exercise most often is a bewildering subject to those who are unfamiliar with the *methods, principles,* and *laws* that govern it. By definition, an exercise is designed to work a specific area of the body and to bring about specific results. Now if you do an exercise wrong, you're still working the body, but you're not working the area intended by the particular instructor or author from whom you are learning. For example, during a hip routine, the hips should be getting nearly 100 percent of the exercise. If this is not happening, then you're doing the routine wrong or improperly. As a result, the hips will exhibit little or no change in appearance.

Exercise shapes the body through a functional friction with gravity. Gravity pulls you down and shortens your body, while proper exercise elongates the body and lengthens it. The principle of elongation is the key to proper exercise and the elimination of cellulite. Proper movement is defined by the principles and laws of body dynamics, which have been illustrated through history by examples such as Galileo's

Leaning Tower of Pisa and Newton's falling apple, defining gravity as the force that tends to draw all bodies in the earth's sphere toward the center of the earth.

Proper exercise stretches and elongates the body away from the center, pulling it upward against gravity. Tension and stress from daily living tend to compress the body, pushing it inward to the center, causing the spine to bend. As a result, the body becomes shorter and older-looking. Proper exercise pulls the body away from the center, stretching the spine, extending the body to its proper height of beauty.

Those of you who deviate from proper form are not working the weak, tight, and fatty areas where cellulite resides but are only enhancing the already strong and flexible areas of your body. *Deviate exercise* is easier and feels more reward-

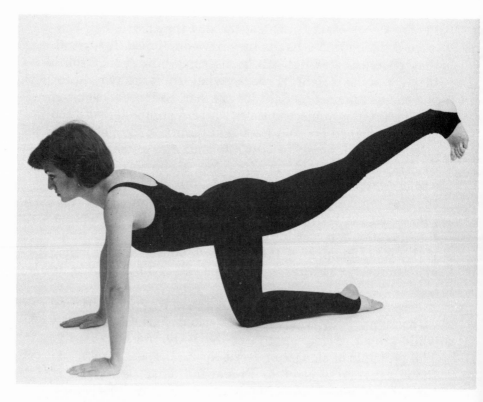

Correct form.

ing at the time of the exercise, but in the long run, it only hurts you. It is natural to back away from pain and to depend on your stronger and more flexible muscles to get you through the exercises. Consciously or unconsciously, everyone does it, and that is why you must study form and technique—so you can observe yourself *objectively*. You must learn that it doesn't matter how high you kick or how low you squat, if some part of your body is deviating. Remember: When you cheat, you're shifting the concentration of the exercise to another part of the body, which defeats the whole purpose of prescribed exercises.

You have to enjoy exercise, or at least the results of what it brings. Your emotional well-being is important, because your attitude can play a large part in your progress. No

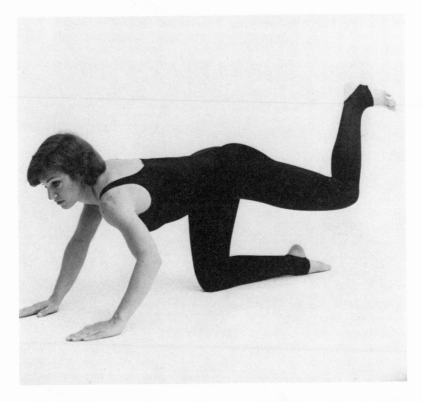

Deviant form.

exercise routine can make your body beautiful if you have a negative attitude toward it. Body language confirms the fact that most people really don't enjoy exercise. They only do it because they know it is good for them. People who dislike exercise and have to force themselves to do it won't be as productive as people who find pleasure in exercise. The pleasure in exercising is found in seeing the results, the fruits of your labor.

People with a negative attitude toward exercise have a tendency to hold their breath while exercising; some simply forget to breathe or hold their breath on purpose. Breathing is a blend of physiology and psychology, and where you draw the line between the two sciences is debatable. Why you hold your breath is also debatable, but most adults who exercise do hold their breath, and it is wrong!

People who hold their breath for too long a period of time cause the body to become fixed and frozen, which makes

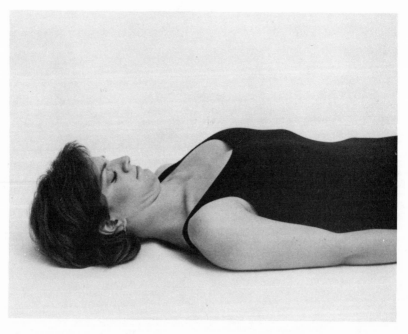

Facial tension inhibits breathing, causing stress to the body.

movement difficult. Breathing and body movement must be coordinated if you are to achieve good results.

The head and neck should always remain neutral and relaxed during the exercise routine to insure proper breathing. The head and neck should never be used to move any part of the body, especially the hips, buttocks, or thighs. The chin and jaw should always be extended away from the throat to insure proper breathing. You should never retract your chin into your throat, because the air from the nose and mouth will not be able to enter or leave the windpipe (larynx/ trachea). The muscles surrounding the face and throat should always be relaxed, to prevent you from holding your breath. When your mouth and throat (larynx) are open, you cannot hold your breath. The cellulite-free-body exercise routine should be done with a slightly open mouth and with your chin extended away from the throat at all times to guarantee proper breathing.

Body language can be read easily by placing a mirror in front of or next to you. This will give you the opportunity to observe and correct your own posture, form, and breathing habits. Breathing habits can be observed by watching your facial expressions. A mirror is a helpful tool, enabling you to see what you look like while you are exercising.

The following body expressions are most commonly used in times of stress during the exercise, and should be corrected immediately to insure proper breathing.

1. Clenching your teeth
2. Pressing your lips together
3. Depressing your chin (double-chin effect)
4. Tensing and contracting your neck muscles
5. Reddening of your face

The cellulite-free-body exercise routine has been designed with special consideration for the "deviate exerciser." The body can be shaped in many different ways by exercise. The manner in which an exercise is performed will determine the degree of success it has on the body. Exercise must be described and articulated, or else the novice will deviate from

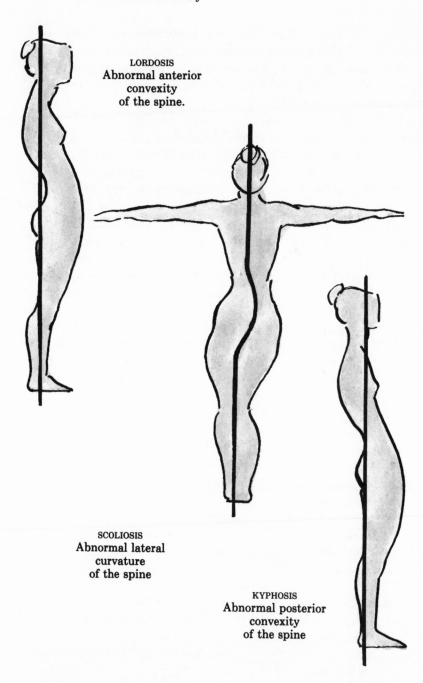

LORDOSIS
**Abnormal anterior
convexity
of the spine.**

SCOLIOSIS
**Abnormal lateral
curvature
of the spine**

KYPHOSIS
**Abnormal posterior
convexity
of the spine**

Postural faults/muscle imbalances.

form and technique. Most exercise routines fail to work because the programs do not take into account the fact that each human body reacts, adjusts, compensates, or deviates in its own way from an exercise. There are four reasons why people deviate from prescribed exercises:

1. They want to make the exercises easier
2. They don't understand the exercises
3. They want to show off
4. They are cheating to compensate for existing imbalances and postural faults.

Number four is the most common reason people cheat while doing their exercises. After years of watching and correcting students in class, I have found that most people deviate from proper form and technique because of postural fault and muscle (connective tissue) imbalances.

The cellulite-free-body exercise routine has been designed to work with your structural imbalances and to make you aware of them. The best method for telling you when you're off center, or cheating, is to observe yourself in the mirror. Of course, a teacher's guidance would be a better way to learn, but for those who cannot afford the time to seek professional help, a mirror will do just fine. The mirror is a subjective reflection of the way you look, because its feedback depends upon how you perceive yourself. Therefore, you must learn to be as objective as possible by following directions to the letter and keeping an open and honest mind. Remember: you are the instructor and you alone are responsible, so don't cheat. Watch your form.

5

The Cellulite-Free-Body Diet Routine

ALMOST EVERYONE IS ON some sort of diet. Every women's magazine you pick up has a new diet to follow, positively promising you that it is the one that will make you thin and beautiful. Being on a diet is the easy part; losing inches around those areas you hate to talk about is not!

Diet is a difficult subject for most people, and one that only a few can deal with honestly. Diet means a lifelong commitment to self-control and self-esteem. Every fat person I have worked with dislikes looking at herself in the mirror while exercising. Looking at yourself is healthy; it gives you perspective on how you're doing. There is nothing wrong with liking yourself enough to take time out of your busy schedule to exercise and watch your diet.

I have three diet principles for you to follow in the fight against cellulite fat. These principles definitely work if you're willing to consume fewer calories and less fat, sugar, and salt!

1. Principle of awareness
2. Principle of substitution
3. Principle of moderation

AWARENESS

The first step in the cellulite-free diet is gaining an understanding about food. Good nutrition starts with becoming aware of what you consume and the nutritional value that you receive. All processed foods have labels that detail the contents of the product, and most offer complete nutritional information. Simply by reading the labels, you can figure out the amount of calories, vitamins, minerals, carbohydrates, protein, and fat you're consuming from that particular product. Reading labels is very important in the fight against cellulite fat.

Most processed foods are filled with refined carbohydrates (sugar and starches), oils, salt, fat (butter, lard, or vegetable shortening), and various preservatives, which can assimilate to create cellulite fat if conditions are right. Being aware of how much butter, salt, oil, sugar, and other ingredients are added to your food makes the difference between supplying your body with needed energy and minerals or overdosing on fat, sugar, and salt. I recommend fresh foods over processed foods, since they are free of added ingredients, are healthier, and have fewer calories.

Being aware of how to prepare your foods is just as important as which foods you use. In cooking, you don't need to use salt as a seasoning. There are other spices, like garlic, black pepper, paprika, and dill weed to name a few, that can be used in the place of salt. When basting your meat, poultry, or fish, you can use water or a little wine instead of butter or gravy. Gravy is 95 percent fat, the fatty juice given off in baking, roasting, or broiling. When you add flour to it, then you're mixing starch and fat together, which will go right to your hips, buttocks, and thighs if you don't watch yourself.

You don't have to be fat to have cellulite! A few of my students are professional models who would be considered skinny, yet they had cellulite in their buttocks and upper thighs. These women do watch their weight, so what were they doing wrong? One, they were not exercising properly, which I corrected; two, they would drink too much coffee with cream and sugar during the day and drink too much wine at night. Wine is very high in natural carbohydrates, because of its sugar (dextrose) content. A half-bottle of wine a night can easily put on two pounds of cellulite within a month if you don't burn it up.

Fat, carbohydrate, or protein in the diet that is not used by the body for energy will be converted into adipose tissue (fat), which can develop into cellulite. It is essential that you be aware of all processed foods and drinks which are filled with salt, sugars, starches, oils, or syrups, whether they are natural as in wine, or added as in soda pop. Either way, they should be avoided.

REFINED CARBOHYDRATES COMMONLY ADDED
TO PROCESSED FOODS:

1. Sucrose: table sugar (sugar cane and sugar beets)
2. Fructose: fruit sugar (sweet fruits and honey)
3. Lactose: milk sugar (found in milk)
4. Glucose: simple sugar (sweet fruits and honey)
5. Maltose: malt sugar (malt and starch)
6. Levulose: fructose (sweet fruits and honey)
7. Dextrose: glucose (grape, corn sugar)

The second step is to have a "blood profile" done once a year to find out if you have too much

1. *Fat* in your diet, which increases the cholesterol and lipid (fat) levels
2. *Carbohydrate* in your diet, which increases the tri-glyceride (sugar) and glucose levels
3. *Salt* in your diet, which increases blood pressure and water retention

The third step is to buy a scale and tape measure, and to become aware of weight and measurement changes by weighing yourself every day and measuring yourself once a week around your upper arms, bust, waist, hips, upper thighs, lower thighs, and calves.

Weights for women.

HEIGHT WITH 2-INCH HEEL SHOES —	SMALL FRAME	MEDIUM FRAME	LARGE FRAME
4'11"	94-101	98-110	106-122
5'0"	96-104	101-113	109-125
5'1"	99-107	104-116	112-128
5'2"	102-110	107-119	115-131
5'3"	105-113	110-122	118-134
5'4"	108-116	113-126	121-138
5'5"	111-119	116-130	125-142
5'6"	114-123	120-135	129-146
5'7"	118-127	124-139	133-150
5'8"	122-131	128-143	137-154
5'9"	126-135	132-147	141-158
5'10"	130-140	136-151	145-163
5'11"	134-144	140-155	149-168
6'0"	138-148	144-159	153-173

A woman's weight will vary during the course of the month, depending on her menstrual cycle. Since hormonal changes in the body can cause loss and gain of water, extracellular fluid, and body weight, weighing yourself is not as accurate as using a tape measure. Water gain is not fat or extra weight, but a normal process in being a woman.

The fourth step begins with not bringing any junk food into the house, because once it is in the house, forget it! Don't make the excuse that you bought it for your roommate, husband, or children. No matter—you ate it! Junk food is one of the main causes of cellulite. A bag of potato chips, chocolate chip cookies, or pretzels washed down with soda pop, beer, or coffee will do you in very nicely. *Junk food* can be defined as foods that are high in sugar, salt, or fat (oil), which add more calories to your diet than their nutritional value. The goal of the cellulite-free-body diet is to get as much *energy* from your food as possible, with as few *calories* as possible.

The fifth step is counting calories. Caloric measurement is the best and easiest way of judging how much weight you're going to gain from a food. Remember, it only takes 3500 calories to produce a pound of body fat. Approximately 15 to 17 calories are needed to maintain each pound of fat the body contains (body weight). For example, if you weigh 110 pounds, then your caloric intake per day should be about 1650 to 2000 calories, depending on your activities (energy output) and body type.

Now if you want to *lose* weight, I recommend an intake of between 800 and 1000 calories per day until you reach the ideal weight for your body type. At that point, cardiovascular (aerobic) exercise, like fast-paced walking or jogging, is recommended so that you can bring your caloric intake up to a normal level without gaining weight. (Aerobic exercise will burn up fat (adipose tissue), but it will *not* get rid of your cellulite unless you correct or neutralize your postural faults while exercising. Keep in mind that it doesn't matter how fast it comes off, but how long it stays away! More people get sick and cheat themselves out of important nutrients from crazy, quick-losing diets. Always check with your doctor before going on any new exercise or diet program. Depending on your age and physical condition, let your doctor know how you're doing regularly for your own protection.

The sixth step is becoming aware of the quantity of liquids you drink in the course of the day. The more liquids you drink, the better. Liquids help keep the "drain" free and flowing. It is also important to drink liquids that are free of refined sugar and salt.

SUBSTITUTION

The principle of substitution is defined as using one food in place of another. Substituting nutritional, low-calorie foods for high-calorie salt-, fat-, and refined-sugar-laden products is the idea.

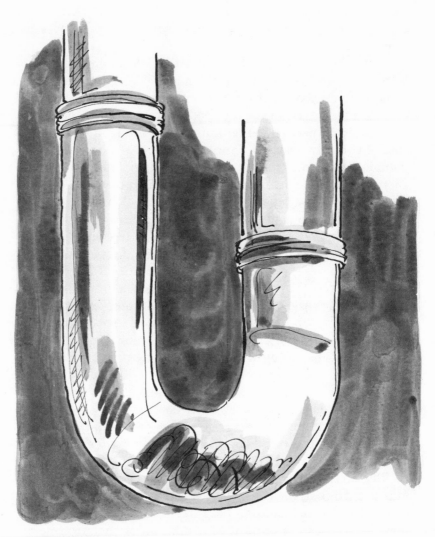

"The Cellulite Trap."

SUBSTITUTION FOODS

1. Polyunsaturated oils for butter, lard, or bacon fat
2. Whites of eggs for cholesterol-filled yolks
3. Skim milk (0% fat) for whole milk
4. Skim-milk cheeses (low fat) for whole-milk cheeses

5. Fish and poultry for meats
6. Lean meat for fatty meat
7. Broiling and baking for frying (cook meat, poultry, fish on a rack so fat can drain off)
8. Water for oil, if possible, when cooking
9. Seltzer water (no salt added) for soda pop
10. Natural fruits and vegetables for refined-sugar and salted snacks (junk food)

No diet can work if you are hungry all the time. You must feel satisfied and fulfilled from your diet or else you will cheat and deviate from it. This is a fact of human nature. By filling yourself up on low-calorie foods and nibbling only on vegetable sticks and citrus fruits, you won't gain as much weight. Furthermore, the vegetables and citrus fruits will act as cleansers in the body, keeping the "drainpipe" open and flowing. For example, a 1-ounce chocolate candy bar has about 147 calories, plus caffeine, fat, and refined sugar, while one medium-size orange has only 71 calories and is packed with plenty of natural energy that is released over a longer period of time, keeping your hunger pains away longer with merely a trace of fat compared to the chocolate bar.

Having a fresh salad instead of a small hamburger for lunch is a good substitution, as long as you don't add too great a quantity of eggs, sliced meats, cheeses, and salad dressing to it—because these ingredients add extra calories, making the salad more fattening than the hamburger. You must count calories and be aware of what you are putting on your salad, for it can make the difference between creating cellulite or getting rid of it! For example, salad dressings are extremely high in calories and fat:

1. Blue Cheese: 76 calories per tablespoon
2. French: 66 calories per tablespoon
3. Italian: 83 calories per talespoon
4. Thousand Island: 80 calories per tablespoon
5. Mayonnaise: 101 calories per tablespoon

Lemon juice or plain vinegar are two good alternatives to

salad dressing, for they contain no dairy cream or oils. Be original and invent your own alternative by trying different spices and low-calorie mixtures.

MODERATION

You can eat anything in *moderation* and get away with it. Most of the time it is not what you eat that gets you in trouble, but how much you eat. Moderation in your consumption of sugar, salt, and fat goes a long way in preventing cellulite. For example, a 1-ounce chocolate bar a day will not hurt you. But add up all the refined sugar that you consume in a day from whatever sources; then you will understand the problem of too much of a good thing! Most of you consume about two pounds of sugar a week (100 lbs. a year), which comes to about one-fourth of your total calories. Three-fourths of the sugar you consume comes in the form of processed foods. Only one-fourth is eaten as pure sugar. For a cellulite-free body, you must exercise moderation in your consumption of processed (packed, canned, frozen) foods. Remember the principle of substitution, and try to substitute fresh foods for processed foods because fresh foods have not been treated with oils, fats, sugar, or salt.

Too much protein, carbohydrate, or fat in your diet is not desirable, either, because what is kept over after building tissue (anabolism) or being burned up as energy (catabolism) will be converted by the chemical processes of the body into fat cells and stored as adipose tissue throughout the body.

Once the fat cells are converted to adipose tissue, they will disperse within the loose connective tissue throughout the body and can surface as the irregular patterns known as cellulite.

6

The Cellulite-Free-Body Exercise Routine

THE CELLULITE-FREE-BODY exercise routine is divided into three levels: beginner, intermediate, and advanced. The routines take between ten and fifteen minutes per session to complete. A beginner is classified as someone who is not familiar with this form of exercise and should take it easy in the beginning to prevent injury. Beginners should practice almost every day to keep the muscles from getting stiff. At the start of any new exercise activity, muscle soreness should be expected and should be treated with massage, hot baths, and balm ointment. Intermediate and advanced people may not need to practice every day—three or four times a week should be enough, because your routines are more extensive than the beginners'.

The key point of these exercises is learning how to position yourself. For example, simply moving your leg up and down will not get rid of your cellulite fat. You must learn to position your leg just right. The cellulite-free-body exercise routine has been scientifically designed to get at the cellulite fat, but if you cheat, or deviate from good form, you will not get rid of it. The improper exercise that you're doing will be a waste of your time. Also, keep in mind that it is not how many repetitions you do or the difficulty of the exercise that matters as much as doing the exercise properly.

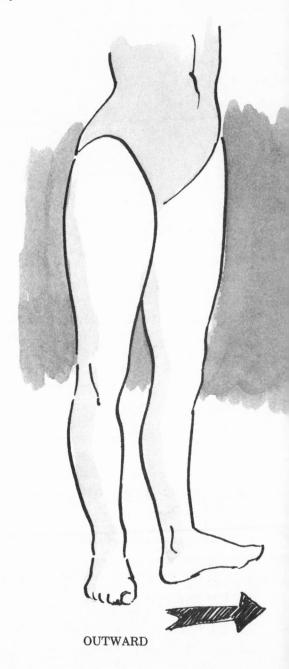

OUTWARD

Rotation at the hip joint.

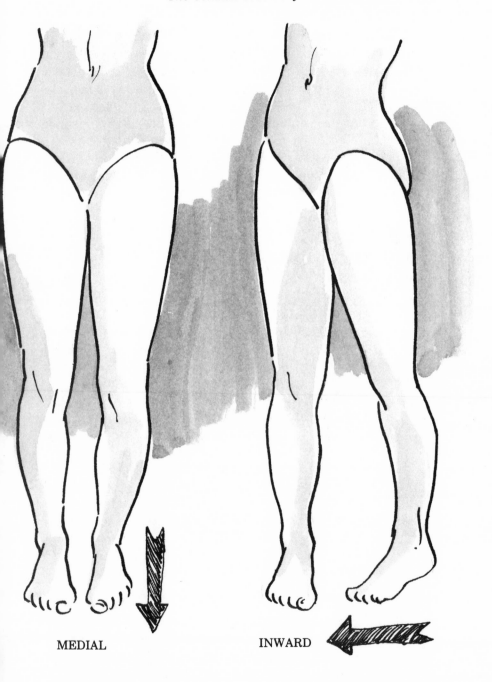

MEDIAL   INWARD

The *pace* you do the repetitions at should be geared to your own individual fitness level. The repetitions can be done as fast as you want, so long as you don't deviate from proper form or hurt yourself in the process by pulling a muscle. Pacing yourself is the safest and easiest way to exercise.

The study of human movement (kinesiology) defines exercise and sport by mechanical means to explain how the body moves. In terms of kinesiology, your leg can rotate three different ways from the hip joint—outward, inward, or medially. Each leg-rotation position works a different part of the hips, buttocks, and thighs. The particular leg rotation you use determines which part of the body will receive the exercise. It is very important to use the correct leg-rotational position that is indicated for each exercise, so that you will receive the proper results.

1. *An outward hip rotation* is defined as rotating the thighbone outward in the hip socket. This particular movement of the thighbone will exercise the *inner part* of the hips, buttocks, and thighs when you move your leg during the prescribed exercise.
2. *An inward hip rotation* is defined as rotating the thighbone inward in the hip socket. This particular movement of the thighbone will exercise the *outer part* of the hips, buttocks, and thighs when you move your leg during the prescribed exercise.
3. *A medial hip rotation* is defined as rotating the thighbone to a neutral position (neither outward nor inward) in the hip socket. This particular movement of the thighbone will exercise the *medial (or lateral) part* of the hips, buttocks, and thighs when you move your leg during the prescribed exercise.

All the prescribed exercises should be done with the feet in a *flexed* position. This position is defined as pushing the heel out and pulling the toes up toward your shinbone (tibia), as opposed to pointing or extending the foot away as is done in ballet and gymnastics. The flexed-foot position is commonly used in karate and modern dance and makes an excellent foot position for getting rid of cellulite. A flexed foot counteracts the effects of wearing high heels by stretching the calf and other lower-leg muscles. Second, it keeps the leg straighter and locks the knee better. And last, there is a stronger tendency for medial and inward-leg rotation with a flexed foot than with an extended-foot position. An inward leg rotation focuses the exercise to the *flank* (female curve) and the *latus* (outer side of the hips, buttocks, and thighs),

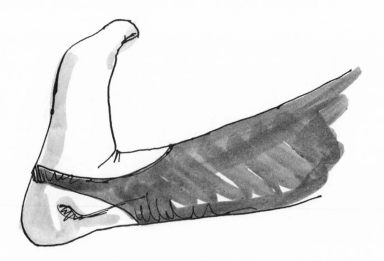

Extended-foot position.

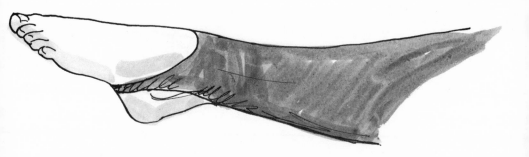

Flexed-foot position.

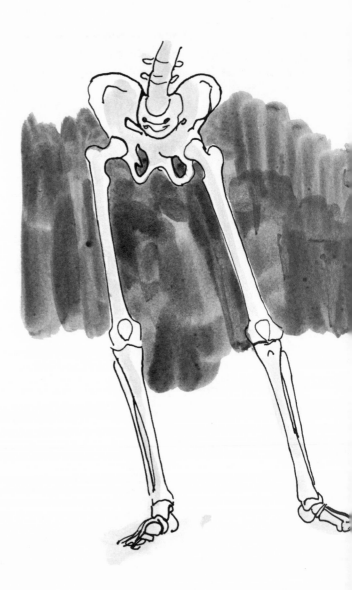

Kinesiological analysis/body positioning.

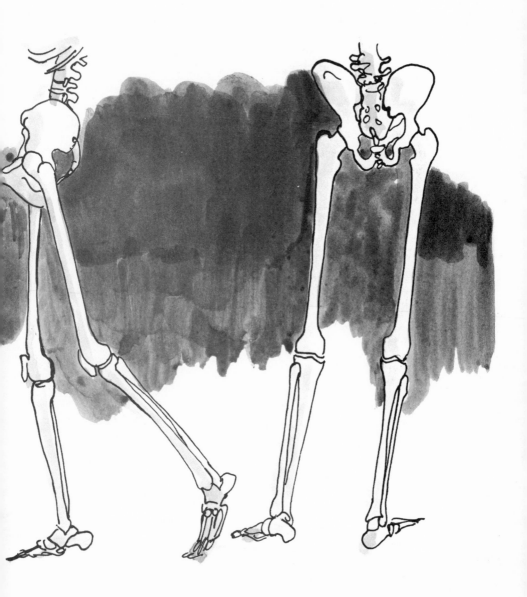

where most of your cellulite generally develops, depending upon the degree of your postural fault (lordosis/knock-knee), while an outward leg rotation focuses the exercise to the inner and frontal areas, which usually don't need as much work. Therefore, I recommend a straight-legged, medial, or inward-leg rotation with a flexed foot whenever possible to eliminate cellulite around the flank and latus area of the hips, buttocks, and thighs.

The novice may think that "kinesiological analysis" is something from outer space. Those who are involved with corrective exercise, sport training, or physical therapy use kinesiology every day in their work. It is the basic language used in explaining and defining human movement. It is about time the novice became aware of kinesiology and the fact that it does matter how you move your body when you exercise.

The exercises in this book are scientifically designed to work, but better yet, they are designed to work at home without an instructor by your side. Learning how to exercise correctly without an instructor is difficult; yet when you use a mirror and follow directions, you can do an excellent job by yourself. *The Cellulite-Free Body* is within your reach, so go for it!

GOOD FORM AND TECHNIQUE MEAN GOOD RESULTS

CORRECT FORM

1. Elbows are straight.
2. Shoulders are square.
3. Hips and buttocks are centered.
4. Raised leg is straight.

DEVIATE FORM

1. Elbows are bent.
2. Shoulders are twisted.
3. Hips and buttocks lean to the side.
4. Raised leg (knee) is bent.

Bending the elbows and leaning to the side cause the raised leg to go higher. This technique is wrong, though, because by cheating, you're shifting the meaning of the exercise from the hip, buttocks, and leg to the lower back and shoulder girdle, deviating from the form and technique which bring good results.

The Exercises

BEGINNER LEVEL—23 EXERCISES

1. straight forward leg raises from a standing position: 5 repetitions (reps.) per leg
2. straight backward leg raises from a standing position: 5 reps. per leg
3. straight sideward leg raises from a standing position: 5 reps. per leg
4. side-to-side trunk bending from a standing position: 5 reps. per side
5. feet-one-foot-apart squats: 5 reps.
6. feet-three-feet-apart squats: 5 reps.
7. back leg raises from on 4s: 10–20 reps. per leg
8. back thigh stretch from on 4s: hold 5 seconds per leg
9. side leg raises with a medial leg rotation from on 4s: 3–5 reps. per leg
10. back leg raises from a semi-handstand position: 1–3 reps. per leg
11. straight sideward leg raises from a semi-handstand position: 1–3 reps. per leg
12. lower leg (calf) stretch for high-heel wearers from a semi-handstand position: hold 1–5 seconds
13. side leg raises with a medial leg rotation from lying on your side: 10 reps. per leg
14. right-angle leg raises from lying on your side: 5 reps. per leg
15. right-angle leg swings from lying on your side: 3 reps. forward and 3 reps. backward
16. right-angle-split leg raises from on your side: 5 reps. per leg
17. inner-thigh leg raises from lying on your side: 10 reps. per leg
18. straight backward leg raises from a prone position: 10–20 reps. per leg
19. straight forward leg raises from a supine position: 5–10 reps. per leg

20. side leg raises with a medial leg rotation from a supine position: 5–10 reps. per side
21. lateral side-to-side with bent knees from a supine position: 5–10 reps. per side
22. right-angle splits from a supine position: 10–20 reps. together and apart
23. saddle sit-ups from a right-angle-split position: 3–5 reps.

INTERMEDIATE LEVEL—29 EXERCISES

1. straight forward leg raises from a standing position: 7 repetitions (reps.) per leg
2. straight backward leg raises from a standing position: 7 reps. per leg
3. straight sideward leg raises from a standing position: 7 reps. per leg
4. side-to-side trunk bending from a standing position: 10 reps. per side
5. feet-one-foot-apart squats: 10 reps.
6. feet-three-feet-apart squats: 10 reps.
7. back leg raises from on 4s: 20 reps. per leg
8. back leg circles from on 4s: 3 times around, reverse direction, per leg
9. back thigh stretch from on 4s: hold 5 seconds per leg
10. side leg raises with a medial leg rotation from on 4s: 5–10 reps. per leg
11. side leg raises with an inward leg rotation from on 4s: 5–10 reps. per leg
12. side and back leg swings from on 4s: 3–5 reps. per leg
13. back leg raises from a semi-handstand position: 3–5 reps. per leg
14. straight sideward leg raises from a semi-handstand position: 3–5 reps. per leg
15. lower leg (calf) stretch for high-heel wearers from a semi-handstand position: hold 5 seconds
16. side leg raises with a medial leg rotation from lying on your side: 20–50 reps. per leg
17. side leg raises with an inward leg rotation from lying on your side: 20–50 reps. per leg
18. side leg circles with an outward leg rotation from lying on your side: 5–10 times around, reverse direction, per leg

19. right-angle leg raises from lying on your side: 5–10 reps. per leg
20. right-angle leg swings from lying on your side: 5 reps. forward and 5 reps. backward
21. right-angle-split leg raises from lying on your side: 5–10 reps. per leg
22. inner-thigh leg raises from lying on your side: 10–20 reps. per leg
23. straight backward leg raises from a prone position: 20–50 reps. per leg
24. straight forward leg raises from a supine position: 5–10 reps. per leg
25. side leg raises with a medial leg rotation from a supine position: 5–10 reps. per leg
26. side leg circles with an outward leg rotation from a supine position: 3–5 times around, reverse directions, per leg
27. lateral side-to-side with bent knees from a supine position: 5–10 reps. per side
28. right-angle splits from a supine position: 10–20 reps. together and apart
29. saddle sit-ups from a right-angle-split position: 5–10 reps.

ADVANCED LEVEL—34 EXERCISES

1. straight forward leg raises from a standing position: 10 repetitions (reps.) per leg
2. straight backward leg raises from a standing position: 10 reps. per leg
3. straight sideward leg raises from a standing position: 10 reps. per leg
4. side-to-side trunk bending from a standing position: 10–25 per side
5. feet-together squats: 5–10 reps.
6. feet-one-foot-apart squats: 10–20 reps.
7. feet-three-feet-apart squats: 10–20 reps.
8. back leg raises from on 4s: 20 reps. per leg
9. back leg circles from on 4s: 5 times around, reverse directions, per leg
10. back thigh stretch from on 4s: hold 5 seconds per leg
11. side leg raises with a medial leg rotation from on 4s: 10 reps. per leg
12. side leg raises with an inward leg rotation from on 4s: 10 reps. per leg
13. side leg raises with an outward leg rotation from on 4s: 5–10 reps. per leg
14. side and back leg swings from on 4s: 10 reps. per leg
15. side leg circles from on 4s: 5 times around, reverse directions, per leg
16. back leg raises from a semi-handstand position: 10–20 reps. per leg
17. straight sideward leg raises from a semi-handstand position: 10–20 reps. per leg
18. side and back leg swings from a semi-handstand position: 5–10 reps. per leg
19. lower leg (calf) stretch for high-heel wearers from a semi-handstand position: hold 5 seconds

20. side leg raises with a medial leg rotation from lying on your side: 50–100 reps. per leg
21. side leg raises with an inward leg rotation from lying on your side: 50–100 reps. per leg
22. side leg circles with an outward leg rotation from lying on your side: 5–10 times around, reverse directions, per leg
23. right-angle leg raises from lying on your side: 10–20 reps. per leg
24. right-angle leg swings from lying on your side: 5 reps. forward, 5 reps. backward
25. right-angle-split leg raises from lying on your side: 10 reps. per leg
26. inner-thigh leg raises from lying on your side: 10–20 reps. per leg.
27. straight backward leg raises from a prone position: 50–100 reps. per leg
28. straight forward leg raises from a supine position: 10–20 reps. per leg
29. side leg raises with a medial leg rotation from a supine position: 10–20 reps. per leg
30. side leg circles with an outward leg rotation from a supine position: 3–5 times around, reverse directions per leg
31. lateral side-to-side with bent knees from a supine position: 5–10 reps. per side
32. right-angle splits from a supine position: 10–25 reps. together and apart
33. right-angle-split circles from a supine position: 5 times around, reverse directions
34. saddle sit-ups from a right-angle-split position: 5–20 reps.

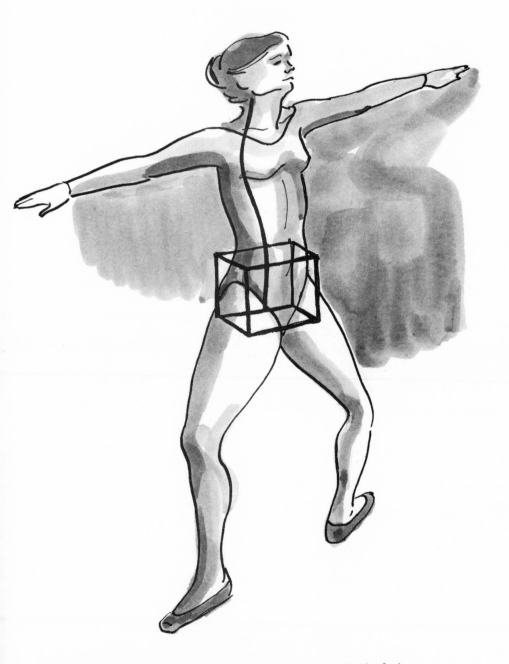

Ballet technique of tucking the pelvis under to neutralize lordosis.

Straight Forward Leg Raises from a Standing Position

Legs and feet together to start, if possible, depending on knock-knee condition.

Arms straight out to the sides, parallel to the ground, slightly below shoulder level.

Torso straight (keep spine and pelvis aligned).

Do not let the pelvis tilt forward—use the ballet technique of tucking the pelvis under to neutralize your lordosis.

1. Right heel in front of you (foot flexed).
2. Raise right leg straight up and down, using a medial leg rotation (see Chapter 6 introduction) to a right angle (90 degrees, or as close to 90 degrees as possible, depending on your flexibility).
3. Keep both legs straight and your knees locked.
4. Keep the left leg stationary.

Beginner level: 5 reps. per leg

Intermediate level: 7 reps. per leg

Advanced level: 10 reps. per leg

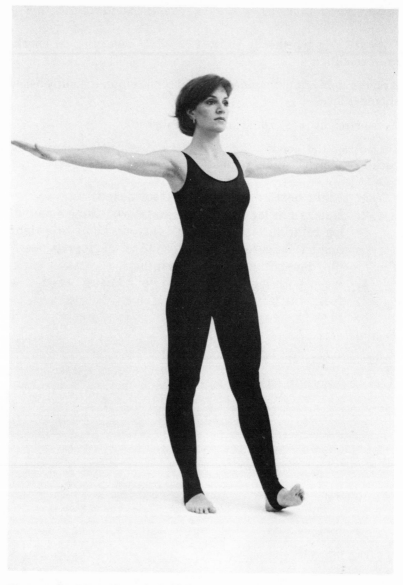

Step 1.   Heel in front; foot flexed.

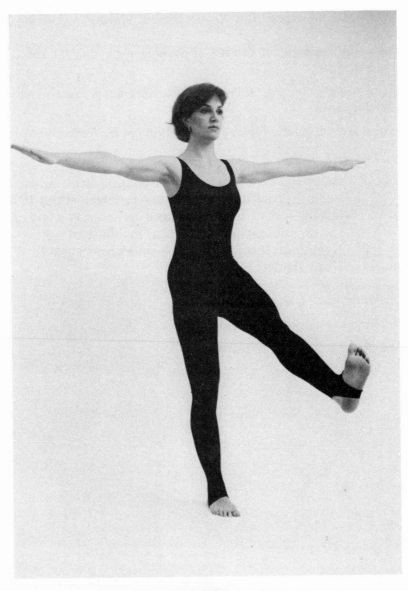

Step 2.   Raise leg straight up and down.

Straight Backward Leg Raises from a Standing Position

Legs and feet together to start, if possible, depending on knock-knee condition.

Arms straight out to the sides, parallel to the ground, slightly below shoulder level.

Torso arched slightly forward (do not lean too far forward).

1. Right foot behind you (foot flexed).
2. Raise right leg straight up and down, using an outward leg rotation (see Chapter 6 introduction) to a level in line with your left knee, or about two feet off the ground depending on your flexibility.
3. Keep both legs straight and your knees locked.
4. Keep the left leg stationary.

Beginner level: 5 reps. per leg

Intermediate level: 7 reps. per leg

Advanced level: 10 reps. per leg

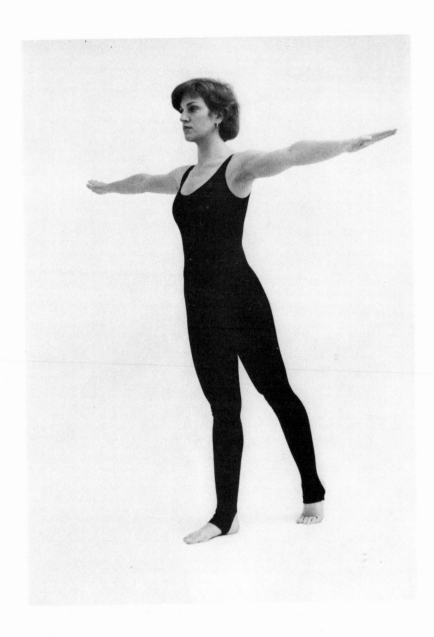

Step 1.　Foot behind; foot flexed.

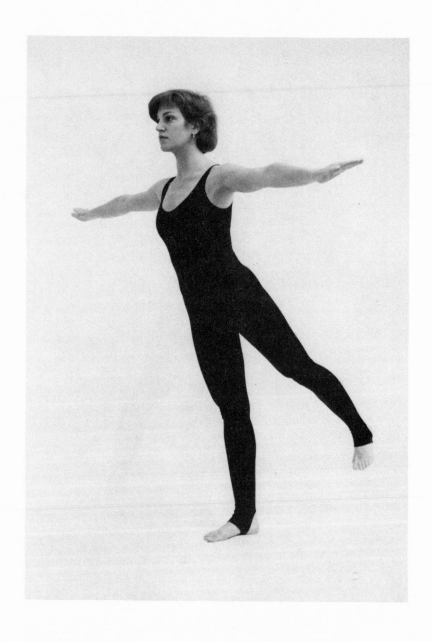

Step 2.   Raise leg straight up and down using outward rotation.

Straight Sideward Leg Raises from a Standing Position

Legs and feet together to start, if possible, depending on knock-knee position.

Arms straight out to the sides, parallel to the ground, slightly below shoulder level.

Torso straight (do not lean sideways).

1. Raise right leg sideways, using a medial leg rotation, to a level in line with your left knee or about two feet away from the ground, depending on your flexibility.
2. Keep both legs straight and your knees locked.
3. Keep the left leg stationary.

Beginner level: 5 reps. per leg

Intermediate level: 7 reps. per leg

Advanced level: 10 reps. per leg

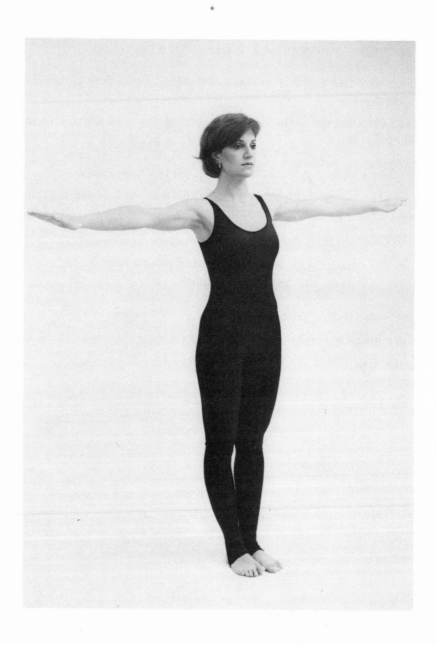

Starting position: feet together, arms outstretched.

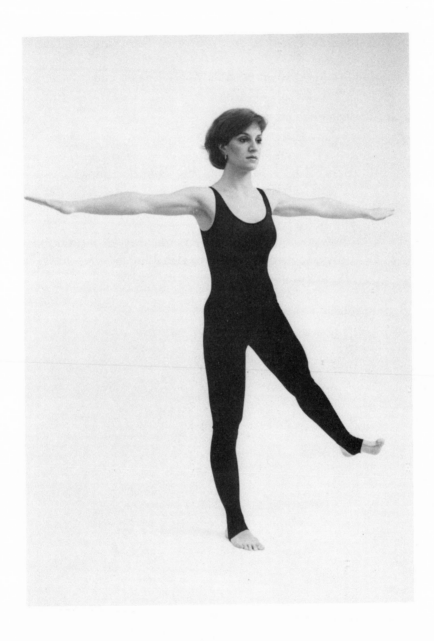

Step 1. Raise leg sideways, using medial rotation.

Side-to-Side Trunk Bending from a Standing Position

Legs and feet together, if possible, depending on knock-knee condition.

Hands clasped behind your head.

Elbows pulling backward, causing the back to arch.

1. Bend side to side from the waist and hips.
2. Alternate right to left.
3. Keep the body centered; do not lean forward; keep the body balanced.
4. How far you can bend depends on your lateral flexibility, so be careful not to strain by moving slowly in the beginning of your repetitions.

Beginner level: 5 reps. per side

Intermediate level: 10 reps. per side

Advanced level: 10–25 reps. per side

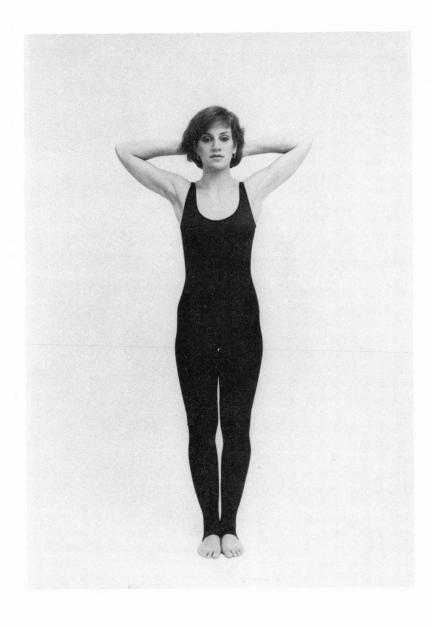

Starting position: feet together, hands behind head, elbows back.

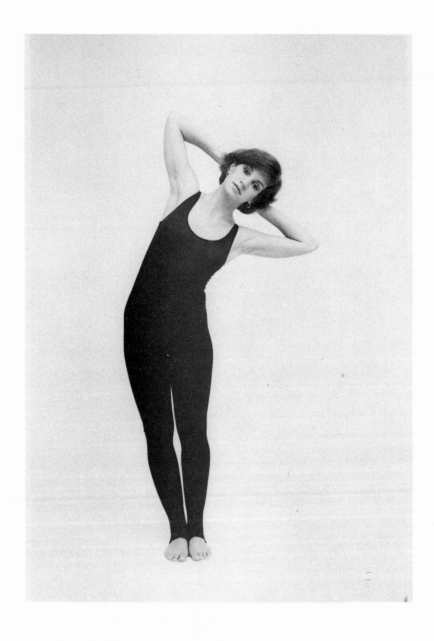

Step 1.   Bend side to side from the waist and hips.

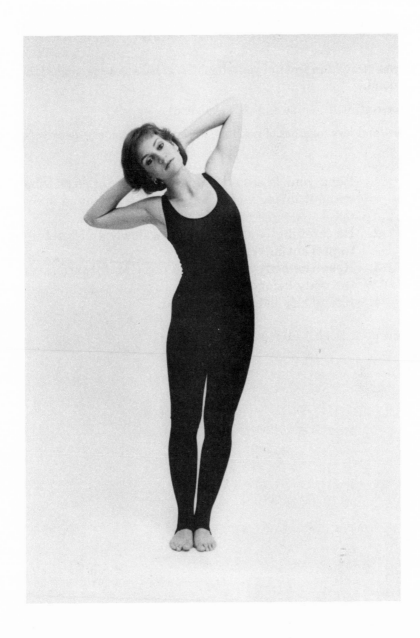

Step 2. **Alternate right to left, keeping body centered.**

Feet-Together Squats

Arms straight in front of you, shoulder-width apart, parallel to the ground.

Torso straight (spine and pelvis aligned).

Feet and legs together, if possible, depending on knock-knee condition.

1. Bend your knees and squat as far down as possible without lifting your heels off the ground and stand up.
2. Be careful of your knees: move slowly and carefully to prevent injury.
3. Keep the body centered; do not lean forward; keep the body balanced.
4. Keep heels flat on the ground.

Advanced level: 5–10 reps.

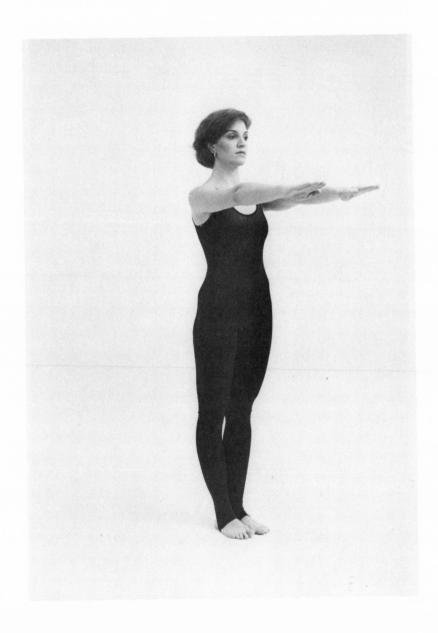

Starting position: feet together, arms out straight in front.

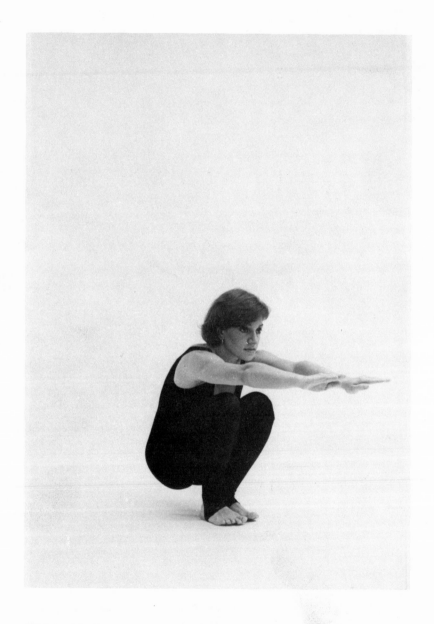

Step 1. Bending knees, squat while keeping heels on ground and body centered; stand up.

Feet-One-Foot-Apart Squats

Arms straight in front of you, shoulder-width apart, parallel to the ground.

Feet one foot apart and parallel.

Torso straight (spine and pelvis aligned).

1. Bend your knees and squat as far down as possible without lifting your heels off the ground and stand up.
2. Keep heels flat down on the ground.
3. Keep the body centered; do not lean forward; keep the body balanced.
4. Be careful of your knees: move slowly and carefully to prevent injury.

Beginner level: 5 reps.

Intermediate level: 10 reps.

Advanced level: 10–20 reps.

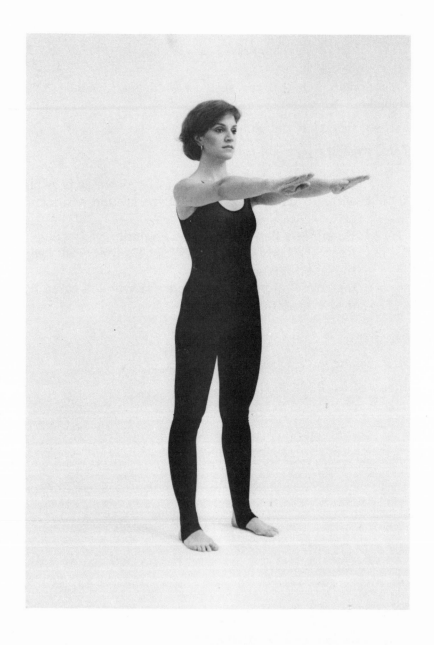

Starting position: feet one foot apart, arms straight out in front.

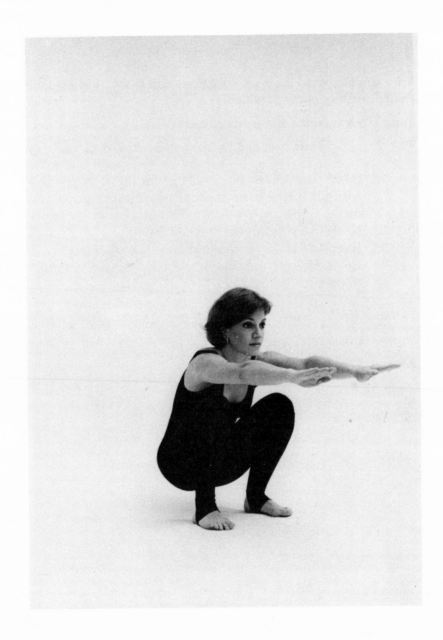

Step 1.   Bending knees, squat while keeping heels on ground and body centered; stand up.

Feet-Three-Feet-Apart Squats

Arms straight out to the sides, shoulder-width apart, parallel to the ground, slightly below shoulder level.

Torso straight (spine and pelvis aligned).

Feet three feet apart; feet and knees turned out 45 degrees.

1. Bend your knees and squat as far down as possible without lifting your heels off the ground and stand up.
2. Keep heels flat down on the ground.
3. Keep the body centered; do not lean forward.
4. Be careful of your knees: move slowly and carefully to prevent injury.

Beginner level: 5 reps.

Intermediate level: 10 reps.

Advanced level: 10–20 reps.

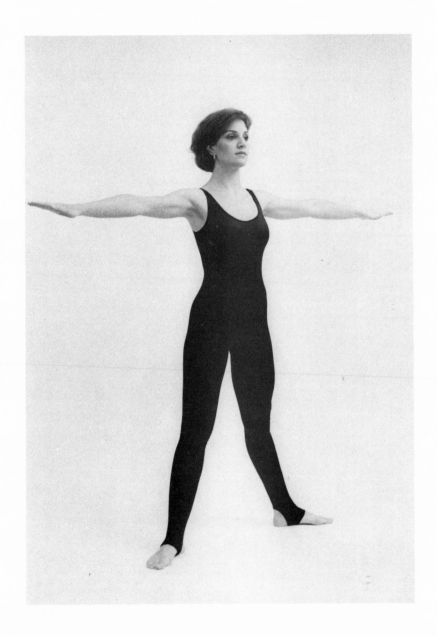

Starting position: feet three feet apart and turned out, arms outstretched.

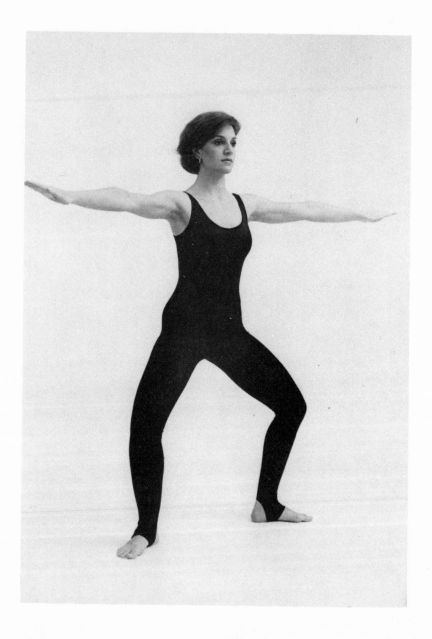

Step 1. Bending knees, squat while keeping heels on ground and body centered; stand up.

Back Leg Raises from on 4s

Kneel down on your hands and knees to begin.

Hands should be shoulder-width apart, no wider.

Palms should be pressed down and kept flat (fingers pointing straight forward).

Knees should be pelvic-width apart.

Supporting knee and leg should be positioned at a right angle and kept stationary, while the active leg does most of the work.

1. Right foot behind you (foot flexed).
2. Raise right leg straight up and down, using an outward leg rotation, to a level which you can achieve without deviating from proper form.
3. Keep elbows straight.
4. Keep back, torso straight; don't move your spine.
5. Keep shoulders square; don't twist.
6. Keep head and neck relaxed; don't move your head.
7. Keep hips centered; don't lean to one side.
8. Remember, the height of your leg raise depends on your hip and leg flexibility, so if you're tight, don't cheat to get your leg higher!

Beginner level: 10–20 reps. per leg

Intermediate level: 20 reps. per leg

Advanced level: 20 reps. per leg

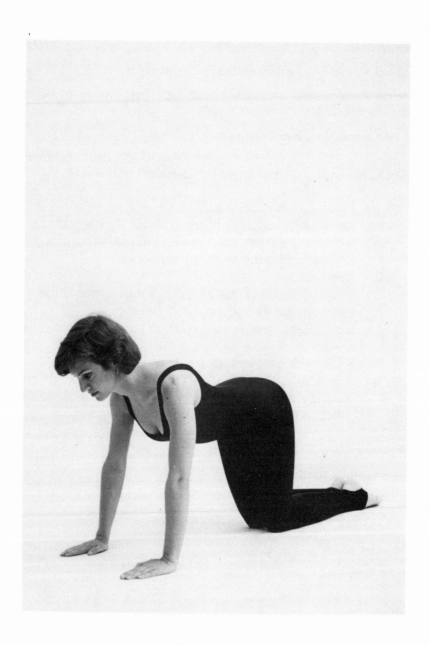

Starting position: kneeling on hands and knees.

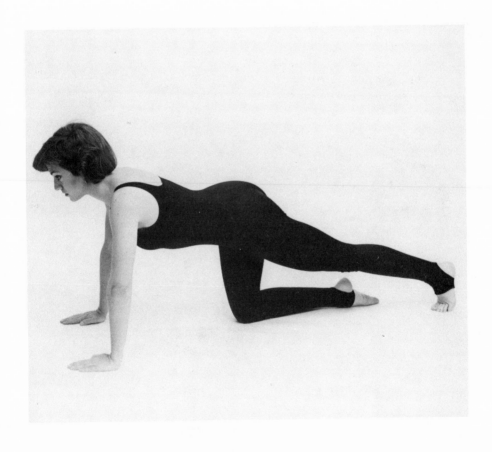

Step 1. Extend leg behind you (foot flexed).

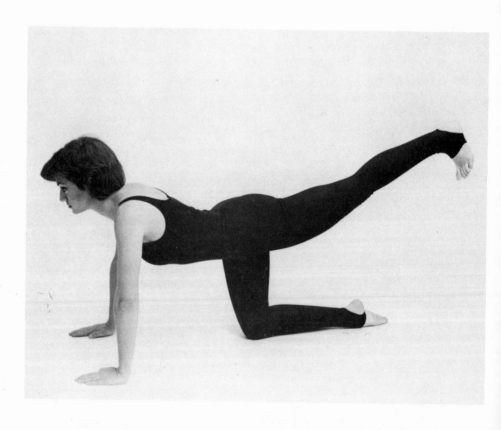

Step 2.   Raise leg using outward leg rotation; keep elbows, torso and back straight.

Back Leg Circles from on 4s

Kneel down on your hands and knees to begin.

Hands should be shoulder-width apart, no wider.

Palms should be pressed down and kept flat (fingers pointing straight forward).

Knees should be pelvic-width apart.

Supporting knee and leg should be positioned at a right angle and kept stationary, while the active leg does most of the work.

1. Right foot behind you (foot flexed).
2. Raise right leg straight up and at a level which you can achieve without deviating from proper form. Then form large circles to the outside; afterward, reverse direction.
3. Keep elbows straight.
4. Keep back, torso straight; don't move your spine.
5. Keep shoulders square; don't twist.
6. Keep head and neck relaxed; don't move your head.
7. Keep hips centered; don't lean to the side.
8. Remember, the height and outline of the circle depend on your hip and leg flexibility, so if you're tight, don't cheat to get your leg higher!

Intermediate level: 3 times around, reverse direction, per leg

Advanced level: 5 times around, reverse direction, per leg

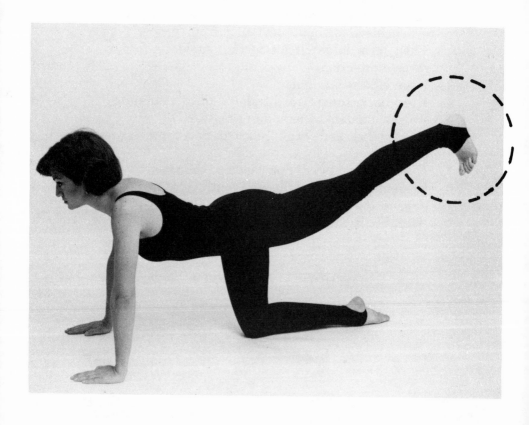

Step 1.   Raise leg straight up and form large circles to the outside; reverse direction.

Back Thigh Stretch from on 4s

Kneel down on your hands and knees to begin.

Hands should be shoulder-width apart, no wider.

Palms should be pressed down and kept flat (fingers pointing straight forward).

Knees should be pelvic-width apart.

Supporting knee and leg should be positioned at a right angle and kept stationary, while the active leg does most of the work.

1. Right foot behind you.
2. Raise right leg straight up as high as possible, and hold.
3. Bend right knee, then bring your right heel as close to your buttocks as possible, depending on your hip and leg flexibility. Hold it there for five seconds.
4. Keep elbows straight.
5. Keep back, torso straight; don't move your spine.
6. Keep shoulders square; don't twist.
7. Keep head and neck relaxed; don't move your head.
8. Keep hips centered; don't lean to the side.

Beginner level: hold 5 seconds per leg

Intermediate level: hold 5 seconds per leg

Advanced level: hold 5 seconds per leg

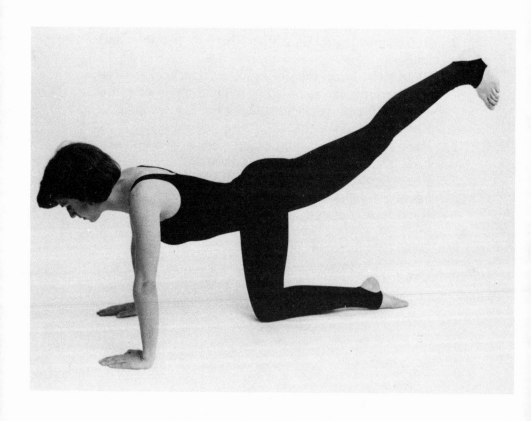

Starting position: leg held out high and straight in back.

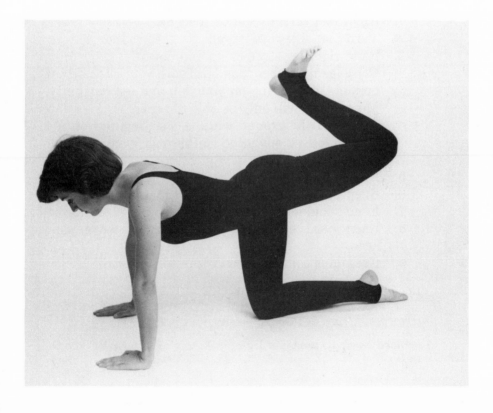

Step 1. Bend knee, bringing heel close to buttocks; hold five seconds.

Side Leg Raises with a Medial Leg Rotation from on 4s

Kneel down on your hands and knees to begin.

Hands should be shoulder-width apart, no wider.

Palms should be pressed down and kept flat (fingers pointing straight forward).

Knees should be pelvic-width apart.

Supporting knee and leg should be positioned at a right angle and kept stationary, while the active leg does most of the work.

1. Right foot directly out to the side.
2. Turn foot sideways, parallel to the ground.
3. Raise right leg straight up and down.
4. Raise leg no higher than level with your shoulders if possible, depending on your hip and leg flexibility. Most of you will only be able to raise your leg a few inches off the ground without cheating, unless you have practiced advanced Hatha yoga, gymnastics, or dance.
5. Keep elbows straight.
6. Keep back, torso straight; don't move your spine.
7. Keep shoulders square; don't twist.
8. Keep head and neck relaxed; don't move your head.
9. Keep hips centered; don't lean to the side.

Beginner level: 3–5 reps. per leg

Intermediate level: 5–10 reps. per leg

Advanced level: 10 reps. per leg

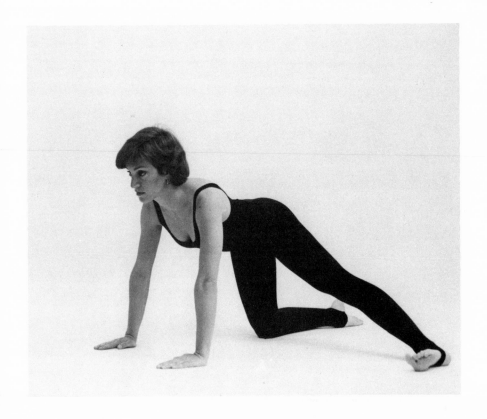

Starting position: foot directly out to side, foot parallel to ground.

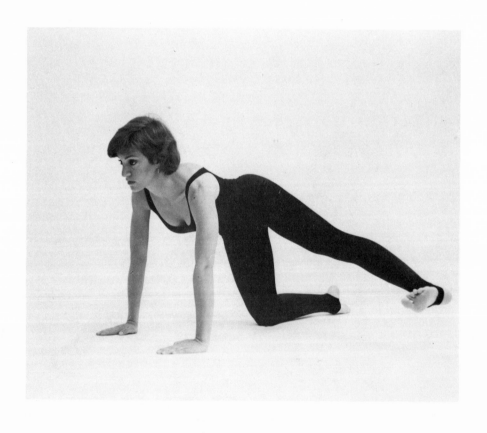

Step 1.   Raise leg straight up and down, no higher than shoulders. Keep elbows, back and torso straight.

Side Leg Raises with an Inward Leg Rotation from on 4s

Kneel down on your hands and knees to begin.

Hands should be shoulder-width apart, no wider.

Palms should be pressed down and kept flat (fingers pointing straight forward).

Knees should be pelvic-width apart.

Supporting knee and leg should be positioned at a right angle and kept stationary, while the active leg does most of the work.

1. Move foot out to the side and rotate it inward.
2. Turn heel up, toes down (flexed-foot position).
3. Raise right leg straight up and down.
4. Raise no higher than parallel to the ground level with your shoulders if possible, depending on your hip and leg flexibility. Most of you will only be able to raise your leg a few inches off the ground without cheating, unless you have practiced Hatha yoga or gymnastics on an advanced level.
5. Keep elbows straight.
6. Keep back, torso straight; don't move your spine.
7. Keep shoulders square; don't twist.
8. Keep head and neck relaxed; don't move your head.
9. Keep hips centered; don't lean to the side.

Intermediate level: 5–10 reps. per leg

Advanced level: 10 reps. per leg

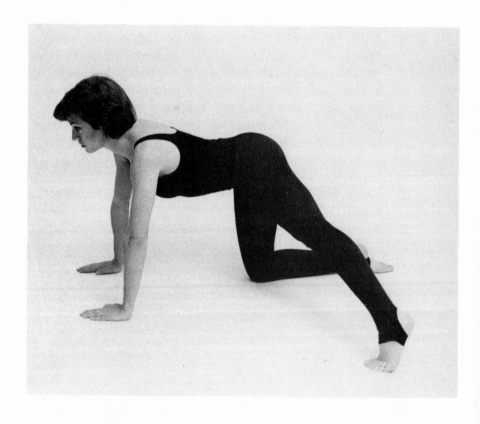

Step 1.   Move foot out to the side and rotate it inward, turning heel up and toes down.

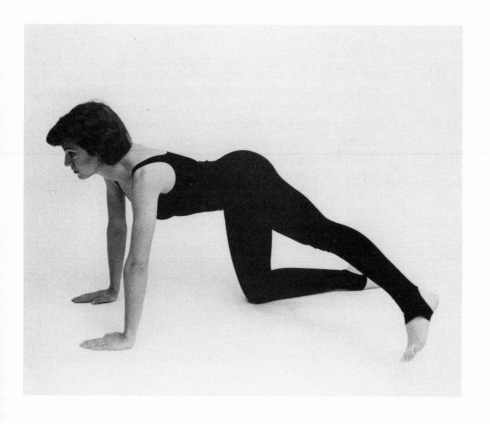

Step 2.   Raise leg straight up and down.

Side Leg Raises with an Outward Leg Rotation from on 4s

Kneel down on your hands and knees to begin.

Hands should be shoulder-width apart, no wider.

Palms should be pressed down and kept flat (fingers pointing straight forward).

Knees should be pelvic-width apart.

Supporting knee and leg should be positioned at a right angle and kept stationary, while the active leg does most of the work.

1. Move right foot out to the side and rotate it outward.
2. Turn heel down, toes up (flexed-foot position).
3. Raise right leg straight up and down.
4. Raise no higher than parallel to the ground level with your shoulders if possible, depending on your hip and leg flexibility. Most of you will only be able to raise your leg a few inches off the ground without cheating, unless you have practiced Hatha yoga, dance, or gymnastics on an advanced level.
5. Keep elbows straight.
6. Keep back, torso straight; don't move your spine.
7. Keep shoulders square; don't twist.
8. Keep head and neck relaxed; don't move your head.
9. Keep hips centered; don't lean to the side.

Advanced level: 5–10 reps. per leg

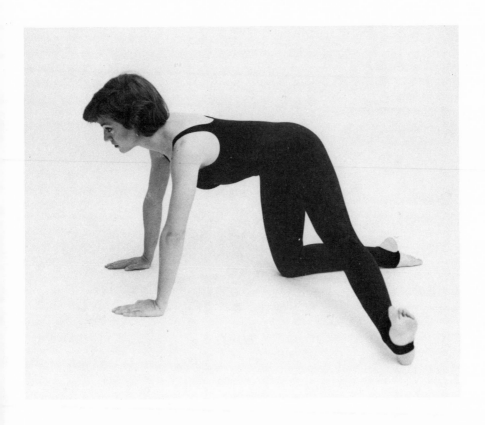

Step 1. Move foot out to the side and rotate it outward, with heel down and toes up.

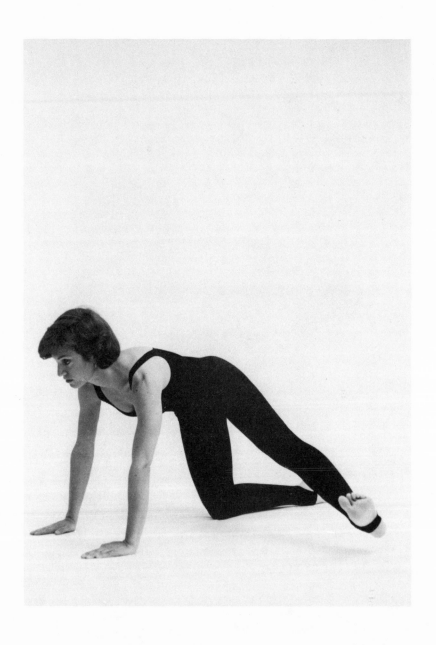

Step 2.   Raise leg straight up and down.

Side and Back Leg Swings from on 4s

Kneel down on your hands and knees to begin.

Hands should be shoulder-width apart, no wider.

Palms should be pressed down and kept flat (fingers pointing straight forward).

Knees should be pelvic-width apart.

Supporting knee and leg should be positioned at a right angle and kept stationary, while the active leg does most of the work.

1. Right foot behind you.
2. Raise the right leg up and hold, then swing right leg forward and back.
3. Keep right leg horizontal as you slowly swing it back and forth.
4. Use medial leg rotation on forward swing and outward leg rotation on backward swing.
5. The level of the right leg from the ground will be determined by your hip, buttock, and leg flexibility; therefore, keep the leg low to insure proper form.
6. Keep elbows straight.
7. Keep back, torso straight; don't move your spine.
8. Keep shoulders square; don't twist.
9. Keep head and neck relaxed; don't move your head.
10. Keep hips centered; don't lean to the side.

Intermediate level: 3–5 reps. per leg

Advanced level: 10 reps. per leg

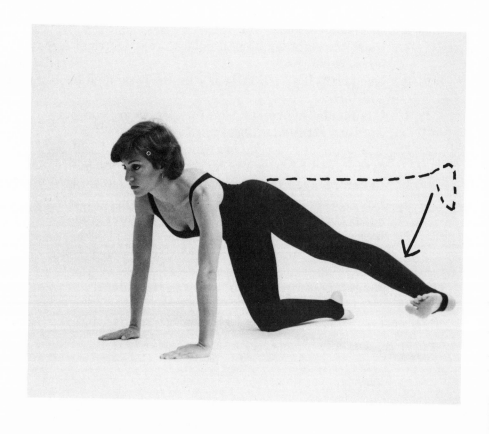

Step 1. Foot behind you. Raise leg and hold.

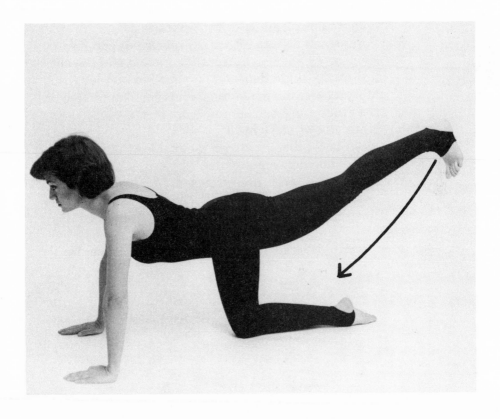

Step 2.   Keeping leg horizontal, swing it back and forth. Use medial leg rotation on forward swing, outward leg rotation on the backward.

Side Leg Circles from on 4s

Kneel down on your hands and knees to begin.

Hands should be shoulder-width apart, no wider.

Palms should be pressed down and kept flat (fingers pointing straight forward).

Knees should be pelvic-width apart.

Supporting knee and leg should be positioned at a right angle and kept stationary, while the active leg does most of the work.

1. Right foot directly out to the side (foot flexed).
2. Raise right leg straight up to a level that you can *hold* without leaning to the opposite side.
3. Form small circles; afterward reverse directions.
4. Remember, the height from the ground and the outline of the circle depends on your hip and leg flexibility; therefore, make the circles small and close to the ground unless you are really flexible.
5. Keep elbows straight.
6. Keep back, torso straight; don't move your spine.
7. Keep shoulders square; don't twist.
8. Keep head and neck relaxed; don't move your head.
9. Keep hips centered; don't lean to the side.

Advanced level: 5 times around, then reverse direction, per leg

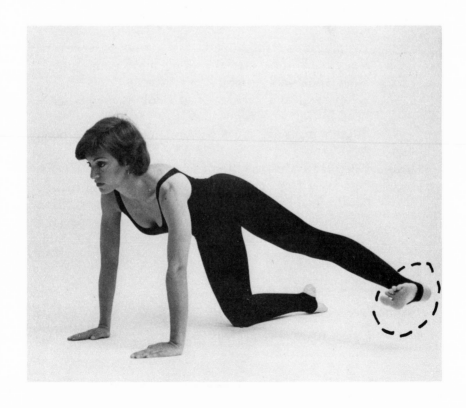

Raise leg out to side (foot flexed) and form small circles. Reverse directions with each leg.

Back Leg Raises from a Semi-Handstand Position

Start from on-4s position, then lift your hips up, straighten your knees, and bring your feet together.

Hands should be shoulder-width apart, no wider.

Palms should be pressed down and kept flat (fingers pointing straight forward).

1. Right foot behind you.
2. Raise right leg straight up as high as possible, then move it down slowly.
3. Keep left leg stationary, left heel flat down if possible.
4. Keep elbows straight.
5. Keep back, torso straight; don't move your spine.
6. Keep shoulders square; don't twist.
7. Keep head and neck relaxed (look at your knees), head in line with arms.
8. Supporting knee must be kept locked; don't bend it.
9. Keep hips centered; don't lean to the side.
10. The level from the ground of the right leg will be determined by your hips, buttock, and leg flexibility; therefore, be careful not to pull a muscle, especially hamstring group, when you raise your leg. Remember to pace yourself.

Beginner level: 1–3 reps. per leg

Intermediate level: 3–5 reps. per leg

Advanced level: 10–20 reps. per leg

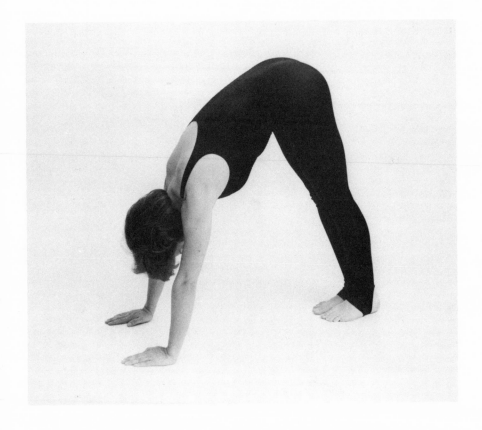

Starting position: feet together, hips up, palms pressed flat.

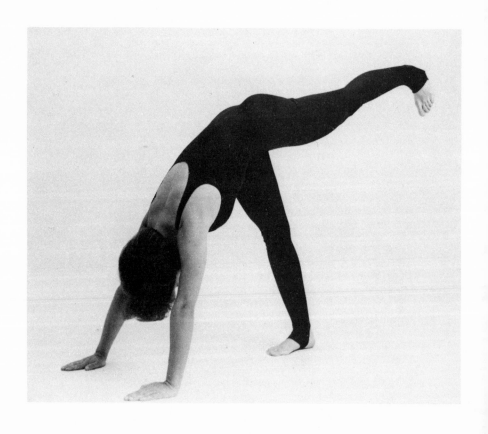

Step 1. With foot behind you, raise leg high, then down slowly.

Straight Sideward Leg Raises from a Semi-Handstand Position

Start from on-4s position, then lift your hips up, straighten your knees, and bring your feet together.

Hands should be shoulder-width apart, no wider.

Palms should be pressed down and kept flat (fingers pointing straight forward).

Feet together, heels together, toes together.

1. Raise right let sideward; move back down. Keep foot flexed.
2. Keep left leg stationary, left heel flat down if possible.
3. Keep elbows straight.
4. Keep back, torso straight; don't move your spine.
5. Keep shoulders square; don't twist.
6. Keep head and neck relaxed (look at your knees), head in line with arms.
7. Supporting knee must be kept locked; don't bend it.
8. Keep hips centered; don't lean to the side.
9. The distance that the right leg can go from the stationary left leg is determined by your right hip and leg flexibility.

Beginner level: 1–3 reps. per leg

Intermediate level: 3–5 reps. per leg

Advanced level: 10–20 reps. per leg

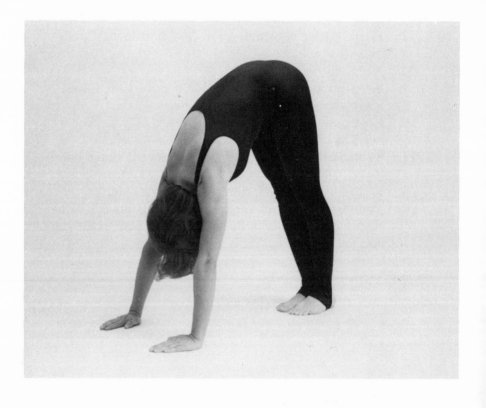

Starting position: feet together, hips up, palms pressed flat.

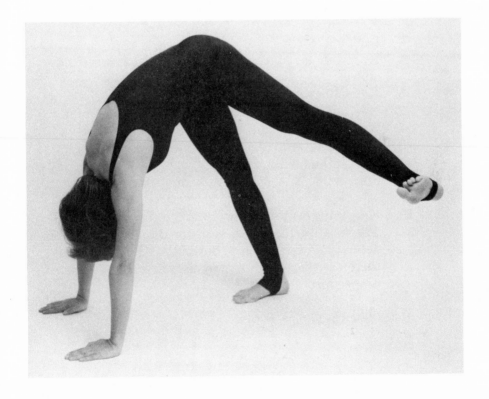

Step 1.   Raise leg sideward, foot flexed, then down slowly.

Side and Back Leg Swings from a Semi-Handstand Position

Start from on-4s position, then lift your hips up, straighten your knees, and bring your feet together.

Hands should be shoulder-width apart, no wider.

Palms should be pressed down and kept flat (fingers pointing straight forward).

1. Put right foot behind you.
2. Raise the right foot up and *hold*, then swing it forward and back.
3. Keep right leg parallel to the ground as you swing it back and forth.
4. Keep left leg stationary, left heel flat down if possible.
5. Keep elbows straight.
6. Keep back, torso straight; don't move your spine.
7. Keep shoulders square; don't twist.
8. Keep head and neck relaxed (look at your knees), head in line with arms.
9. Supporting knee must be kept locked; don't bend it.
10. Keep hips centered; don't lean to the side.
11. The level of the right leg from the ground will be determined by your hip, buttock, and leg flexibility; therefore, keep the leg low as you swing to insure proper form.

Advanced level: 5–10 reps. per leg

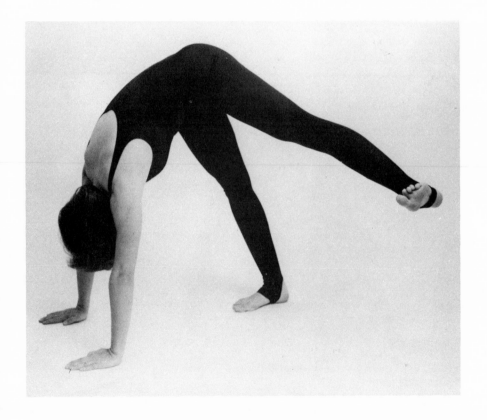

Step 1.   Foot behind you, raise leg up and hold.

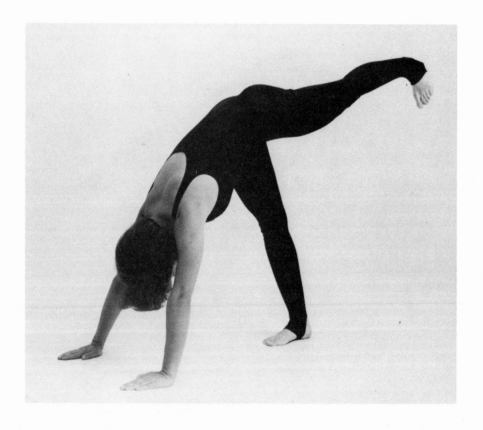

Step 2.   Swing leg back and forth while keeping it parallel to ground.

Lower Leg (calf) Stretch for High-Heel Wearers from a Semi-Handstand Position

Start from on-4s position, then lift your hips and knees off the ground.

Straighten your knees and bring your feet together.

Hands should be shoulder-width apart, no wider.

Palms should be pressed down and kept flat (fingers pointing straight forward).

Feet together, heels together, toes together.

1. Try to press your heels down flat against the ground.
2. Hold your heels against the ground, or as close to the ground as possible, depending on your flexibility.
3. Keep elbows straight.
4. Keep back, torso straight; don't move your spine.
5. Keep shoulders square; don't twist.
6. Keep head kept in line with arms (look at your knees).
7. Keep knees locked, both legs straight.
8. Keep hips centered; don't lean to the side.

Beginner level: hold 1–5 seconds

Intermediate level: hold 5 seconds

Advanced level: hold 5 seconds

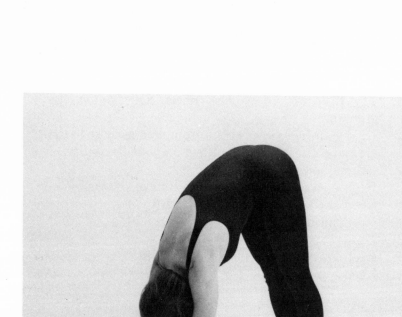

Step 1.   Try to press heels down flat against the ground.

Side Leg Raises with a Medial Leg Rotation from Lying on Your Side

Lie on left side, body elongated laterally.

Legs together, ankles and feet together, with both knees locked and legs perfectly straight.

Bend left elbow at 45-degree angle, place left hand by the side of your head.

Support your head with your left hand.

Place right palm in front of you and keep it flat (don't move it).

Keep right arm straight (do not bend right elbow).

1. Raise right leg straight up and down, using a medial leg rotation (see Chapter 6 introduction) as high as possible.
2. Pelvis and hips should be kept centered throughout the exercise to insure that the medial leg muscles (tensor fasciae latae and gluteus minimus) receive the work.
3. Keep left leg (bottom leg) straight and stationary.
4. Remember to pace yourself so as to prevent injury

Beginner level: 10 reps. per leg

Intermediate level: 20–50 reps. per leg

Advanced level: 50–100 reps. per leg

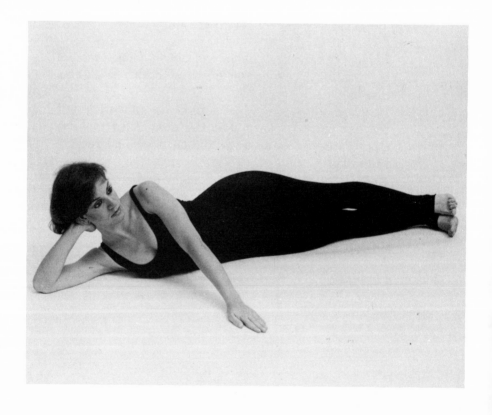

Starting Position: lie on one side, feet together.

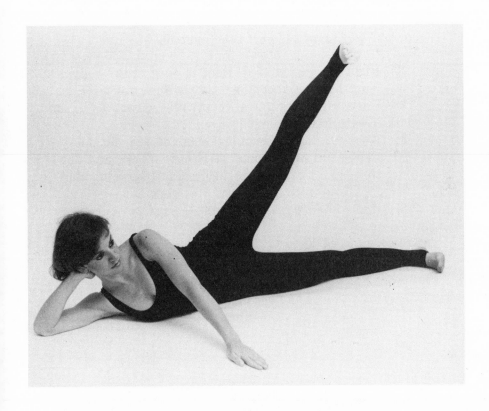

Step 1. Raise leg on opposite side straight up and down, using a medial leg rotation.

Side Leg Raises with an Inward Leg Rotation from Lying on Your Side

Lie on left side, body elongated laterally.

Legs together, ankles and feet together, with both knees locked and legs perfectly straight.

Bend left elbow at 45-degree angle; place left hand by the side of your head.

Support your head with left hand.

Place right palm down in front of you and keep it flat (don't move it).

Keep right arm straight (do not bend right elbow).

1. Right leg angled 45 degrees in *back* of the body.
2. Turn heel up, toes down (flexed-foot position).
3. Raise right leg straight up and down, using an inward leg rotation.
4. Keep left leg (bottom leg) straight and stationary.
5. Pelvis and hips should be *tilted forward* and down throughout exercise to insure that the outer flank, hips, and buttocks receive the work.
6. Remember to pace yourself so as to prevent injury.

Intermediate level: 20–50 reps. per leg

Advanced level: 50–100 reps. per leg

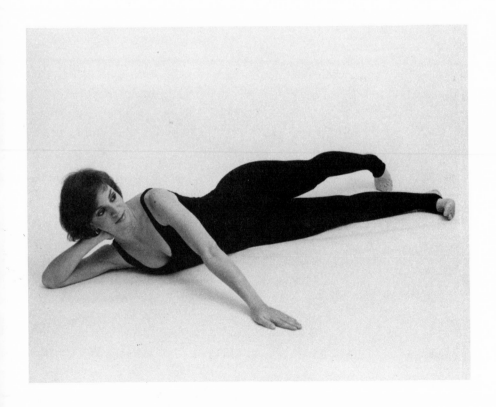

Step 1. Leg angled 45 degrees back, heel up and toes down.

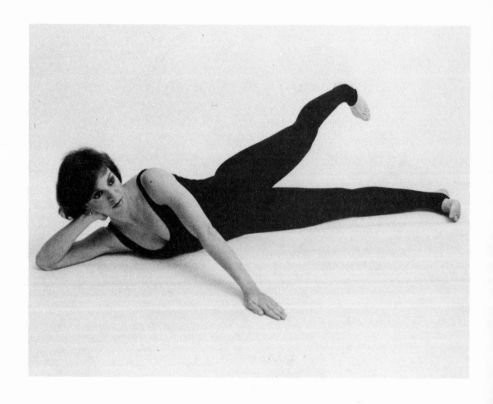

Step 2.   Raise leg straight up and down, using an inward leg rotation.

Side Leg Circles with an Outward Leg Rotation from Lying on Your Side

Lie on left side, body elongated laterally.

Legs together, ankles and feet together, with both knees locked and legs perfectly straight.

Bend left elbow at 45-degree angle; place left hand by the side of your head.

Support your head with left hand.

Place right palm down in front of you and keep it flat (don't move it).

Keep right arm straight (do not bend right elbow).

1. Raise right leg straight up and rotate it outward to a level you can hold, then lower and circle it around, keeping the leg rotated outward.
2. Keep the right leg perfectly straight as you circle it (don't bend your knee).
3. Keep left leg (bottom leg) straight and stationary.

Intermediate level: 5–10 times around, reverse direction, per leg

Advanced level: 5–10 times around, reverse direction, per leg

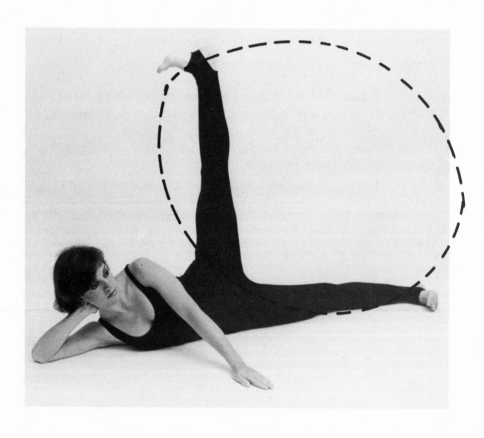

Step 1.   Raise leg straight up, rotate it outward, then lower and circle.

Right-Angle Leg Raises from Lying on Your Side

Lie on left side, body elongated laterally.

Legs together, ankles and feet together, with both knees locked and legs perfectly straight.

Bend left elbow at 45-degree angle; place left hand by the side of your head.

Support your head with left hand.

Place right palm down in front of you and keep it flat (don't move it).

Keep right arm straight (do not bend right elbow).

Move both legs together to a right angle, L-position in front of you.

1. Raise right leg straight up and down; using a medial leg rotation (foot flexed).
2. How high the leg goes depends on your flexibility; as long as you do the exercise correctly, it doesn't matter how high it goes.
3. Do not let your hips fall backward. Tuck the pelvis under and try to center and balance yourself. If you do the leg raises with the hips falling backward, you will not get at the cellulite fat! You must use the "tuck the pelvis under" technique to compensate for a forward pelvic tilt or lordosis condition.
4. Keep the left leg (bottom leg) straight and stationary.

Beginner level: 5 reps. per leg

Intermediate level: 5–10 reps. per leg

Advanced level: 10–20 reps. per leg

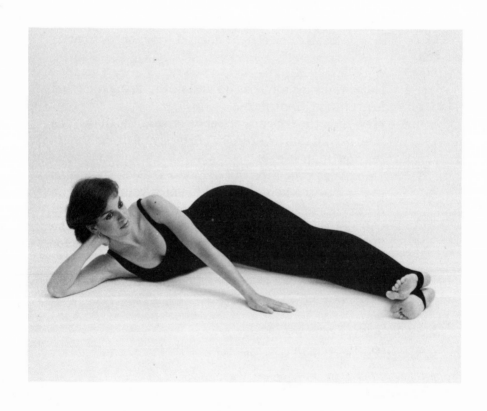

Starting position: lie on one side in L-position, feet together, hand supporting head.

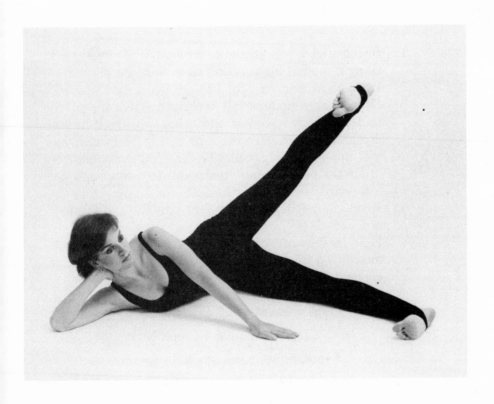

Step 1. Raise leg on opposite side straight up and down, using a medial leg rotation (foot flexed).

Right-Angle Leg Swings from Lying on Your Side

Lie on left side, body elongated laterally.

Legs together, ankles and feet together, with both knees locked and legs perfectly straight.

Bend left elbow at 45-degree angle; place left hand by the side of your head.

Support your head with left hand.

Place palm down in front of you and keep it flat (don't move it).

Move both legs together to a right-angle, L position in front of you.

1. Swing right leg straight forward and backward, using a medial leg rotation (foot flexed).
2. Keep right arm straight (do not bend right elbow).
3. Do not let your hips fall backward. Tuck the pelvis under and try to center and balance yourself. If you do the leg raises with the hips falling backward, you will not get at the cellulite fat! You must use the "tuck the pelvis under" technique to compensate for a forward pelvic tilt or lordosis condition.
4. Keep the left leg (bottom leg) straight and stationary.
5. How far forward or backward the leg goes depends on your flexibility; as long as you do the exercise correctly, it doesn't matter how far the leg goes.

Beginner level: 3 reps. forward and 3 reps. backward

Intermediate level: 5 reps. forward and 5 reps. backward

Advanced level: 5 reps. forward and 5 reps. backward

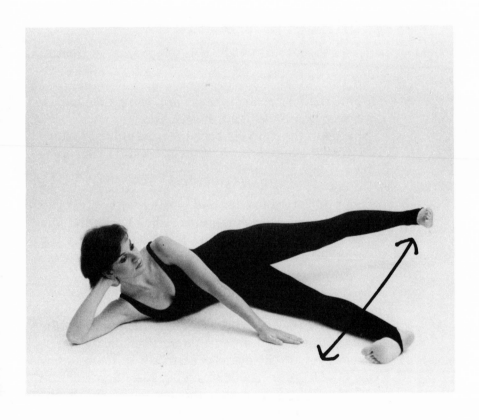

Step 1. Swing leg forward and backward, using medial leg rotation.

Right-Angle-Split Leg Raises from Lying on your Side

Lie on left side, body elongated laterally.

Legs together, ankles and feet together, with both knees locked, and legs perfectly straight.

Bend left elbow at 45-degree angle; place left hand by the side of your head.

Support your head with left hand.

Place right palm in front of you down and keep it flat (don't move it).

Keep right arm straight (do not bend right elbow).

Move both legs together to a right angle, L-position in front of you.

1. Swing right leg straight backward, using a medial leg rotation, and *hold* (split position).
2. Now leave the right leg back near the ground and try to raise it up and down without bending your knee (flexed-foot position).
3. Do not let your hips fall backward. Tuck the pelvis under and try to center and balance yourself. If you do the leg raises with the hips falling backward, you will not get at the cellulite fat! You must use the "tuck the pelvis under" technique to compensate for a forward pelvic tilt or lordosis condition.
4. Keep the left leg (bottom leg) straight and stationary.
5. How high the leg goes up or how far down to the ground the leg goes depends on your flexibility; as long as you do the exercise correctly, it doesn't matter how high or how low the leg goes. Some of you will be only able to lift the leg one inch off the ground, and that's okay, because it is a beginning.

Beginner level: 5 reps. per leg

Intermediate level: 5–10 reps. per leg

Advanced level: 10 reps. per leg

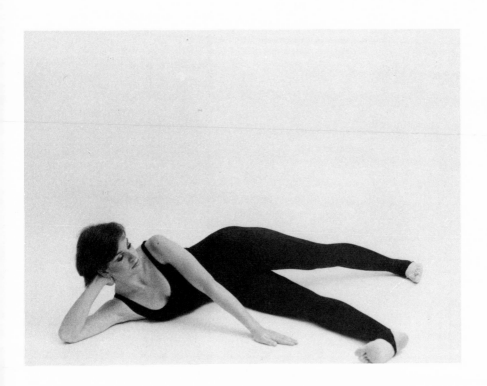

Step 1.   Swing leg backward and hold.

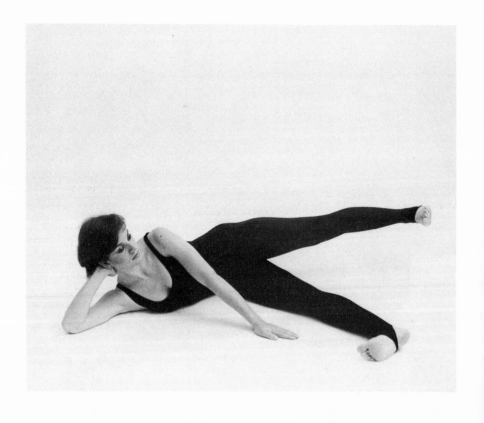

Step 2.   Leg still back, raise it from the ground, leg straight, then down.

Inner-Thigh Leg Raises from Lying on Your Side

Lie on right side, body elongated laterally.

Bend right elbow at a 45-degree angle; place right hand by the side of your head.

Support your head with right hand.

Place left palm in front of you down, and keep it flat (don't move it).

Keep left arm straight (do not bend left elbow).

Bend left knee.

Place left foot in front of the right thigh, or if you're too tight, then the right knee.

Keep left foot flat down, and keep left leg stationary.

1. With locked knee, raise right leg up and down, using a medial leg rotation.
2. Right foot should be parallel to the ground as you lift it.
3. The height of the leg raise depends on your hip, buttock, and leg flexibility. For most of you, twelve inches off the ground will be good.

Beginner level: 10 reps. per leg

Intermediate level: 10–20 reps. per leg

Advanced level: 10–20 reps. per leg

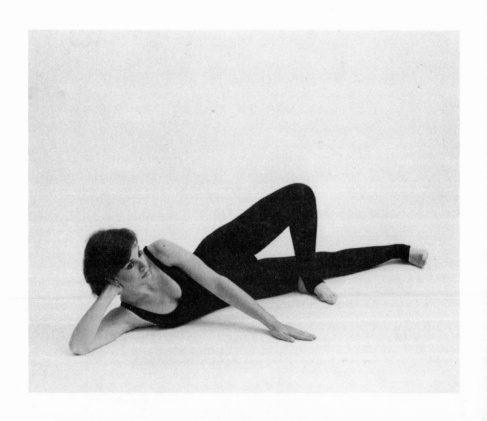

Starting position: lie on one side, support head with hand, opposite arm straight in front, foot crossed in front of thigh on floor.

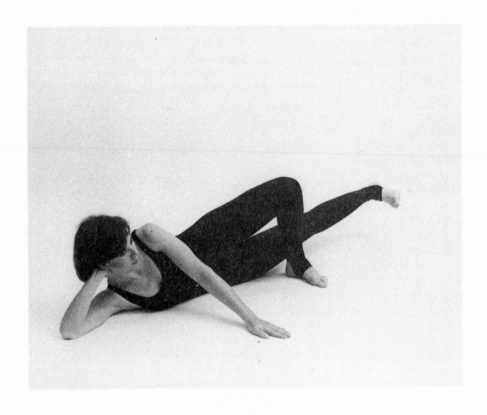

Step 1. Raise leg nearest floor up and down, foot parallel to the ground.

Straight Backward Leg Raises from a Prone Position

Lie down on your stomach to start.

Bend your elbows and place your palms flat down on the ground in front of you, with your chin resting on top of your hands.

Stretch chin forward for good breathing (don't move chin).

1. Raise right leg up and down as high as possible, using a medial leg rotation with knee locked and leg perfectly straight (flexed-foot position).
2. Keep left leg stationary and straight.
3. Remember to pace yourself.

Beginner level: 10–20 reps. per leg

Intermediate level: 20–50 reps. per leg

Advanced level: 50–100 reps. per leg

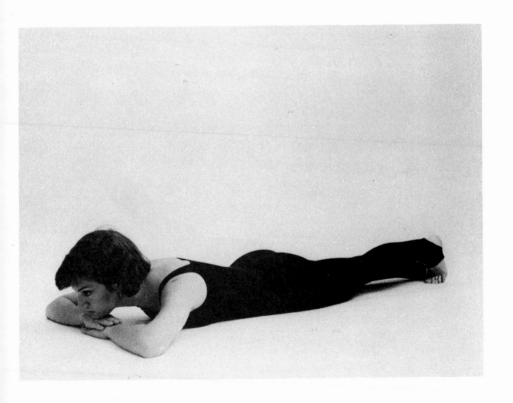

Starting position: lie on stomach, chin resting on top of hands.

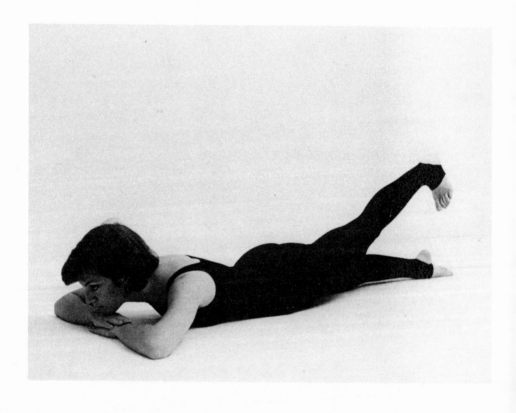

Step 1.   Leg straight, raise leg up and down as high as possible.

Straight Forward Leg Raises from a Supine Position

Lie down on your back to start.

Move arms straight out to the sides (cross position).

Palms should be kept flat down.

Press lower back down (lumbar flattening technique).

Bend left knee; put left foot flat down on the ground, left heel as close to buttocks as possible.

1. Raise right leg up and down to 90 degrees or as high as possible, using a medial leg rotation (foot flexed).
2. Raise only to a 90-degree angle, no further, or else your back will come off the ground.
3. Keep right leg perfectly straight by locking your knee.
4. Keep the left leg stationary, foot flat down.
5. Keep both sides of your buttocks down on the ground (lumbar flattening).
6. Keep head down and relaxed—keep chin away from your throat.
7. Keep torso, back straight; do not twist body.

Beginner level: 5–10 reps. per leg

Intermediate level: 5–10 reps. per leg

Advanced level: 10–20 reps. per leg

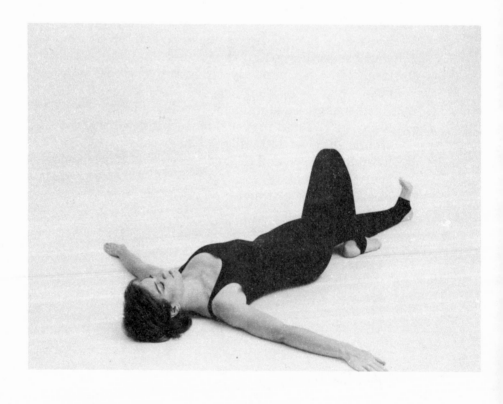

Starting position: lie on back, arms out to side, bend one leg with heel close to buttocks.

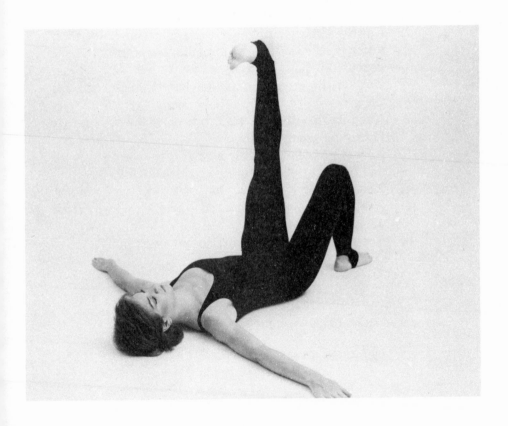

Step 1. Raise opposite leg to 90 degrees and hold, foot flexed.

Side Leg Raise with a Medial Leg Rotation from a Supine Position

Lie down on your back to start.

Move arms straight out to the sides (cross position).

Palms should be kept flat down.

Press lower back down (lumbar flattening technique).

Bend left knee; put left foot flat down on the ground, left heel as close to buttocks as possible.

1. Raise right leg up to a right angle and *hold*, then lower it sideways, using a medial leg rotation and a flexed-foot position, only as far as left buttock can stay on the ground; don't let left buttock come off the ground.
2. Keep both sides of your buttocks down (lumbar flattening technique).
3. Keep right leg perfectly straight as you raise it up and down.
4. Keep left leg stationary, foot flat down.
5. Keep head down and relaxed—keep chin away from your throat.
6. Keep torso, back straight; do not twist body.

Beginner level: 5–10 reps. per leg

Intermediate level: 5–10 reps. per leg

Advanced level: 10–20 reps. per leg

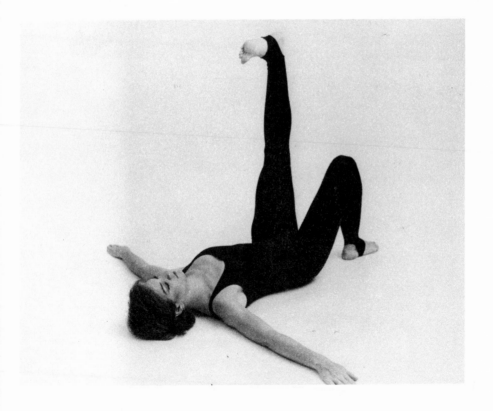

Step 1. Raise leg to right angle and hold.

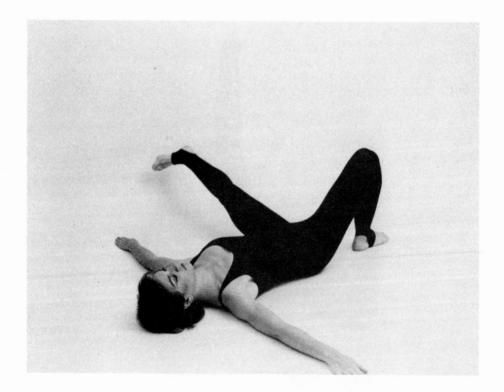

Step 2. Lower leg sideways.

Side Leg Circles with an Outward Leg Rotation from a Supine Position

Lie down on your back to start.

Move arms straight out to the sides (cross position).

Palms should be kept flat down.

Press lower back down (lumbar flattening technique).

Bend left knee; put left foot flat down on the ground, left heel as close to buttocks as possible.

1. Raise right leg up to a right angle and *hold*, then lower and circle around, using an outward leg rotation and a flexed-foot position, only as far as left buttock can stay on the ground; don't let left buttock come off the ground.
2. Keep both sides of your buttocks down (lumbar flattening technique).
3. Keep right leg perfectly straight as you circle it around.
4. Keep left leg stationary, foot flat down.
5. Keep head down and relaxed—keep chin away from your throat.
6. Keep torso, back straight; do not twist body.

Intermediate level: 3–5 times around, reverse directions, per leg

Advanced level: 3–5 times around, reverse directions, per leg

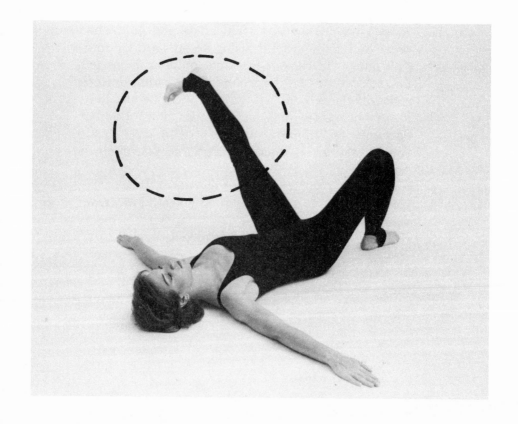

Step 1.   From right angle, lower leg and circle it around.

Lateral Side to Side with Bent Knees from a Supine Position

Lie down on your back to start.

Move arms straight out to the sides (cross position).

Palms should be kept flat down.

Press upper back (shoulder blades) down.

1. Bend (tuck) both knees as close as you can into your chest.
2. Press flexed feet and knees together; do not let knees come apart.
3. Move bent knees side to side.
4. Feet do not touch floor when you alternate *laterally right to left*; only the knees, thighs, buttocks, and hips do.
5. Keep head down and relaxed—keep chin away from your throat.
6. Keep upper back (shoulder blades) stationary, as the lower back *twists* with the lateral movement of the knees.
7. Try to lift from the ground with the bottom knee first, because it will help you to keep your knees together.

Beginner level: 5–10 reps. per side

Intermediate level: 5–10 reps. per side

Advanced level: 5–10 reps. per side

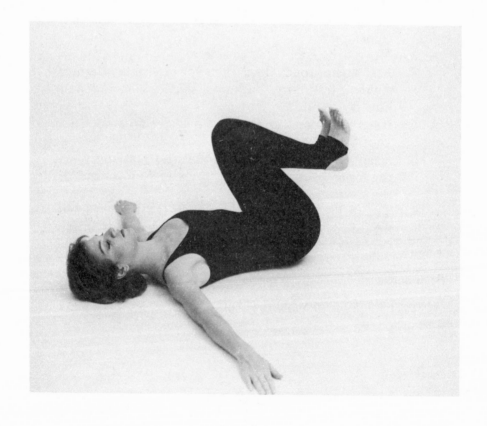

Starting Position: lie on back, tuck knees to chest, arms out to sides.

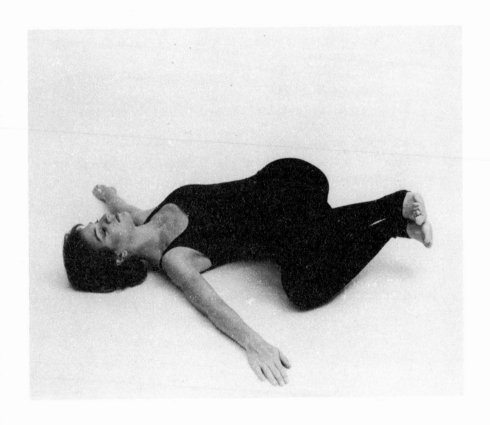

Step 1.   Feet and knees together, move bent legs side to side.

Right-Angle Splits from a Supine Position

Lie down on your back to start.

Move arms straight out to the sides (cross position).

Palms should be kept flat down.

Press lower back down (lumbar flattening technique).

1. Raise both legs together with locked knees straight up to a right angle or as close to 90 degrees as possible, while still keeping the lower back flat on the ground, and *hold*; then move both legs apart and back together, using a medial leg rotation with flexed feet.
2. Try to keep both legs straight and the lower back flat on the ground.
3. Keep head down and relaxed—keep chin away from your throat.
4. Keep torso, back straight; do not twist body.
5. The distance apart of the legs in the split will be determined by your hip and leg flexibility, so be careful not to split your legs too far apart so as to prevent injury.

Beginner level: 10–20 reps. together and apart

Intermediate level: 10–20 reps. together and apart

Advanced level: 10-25 reps. together and apart

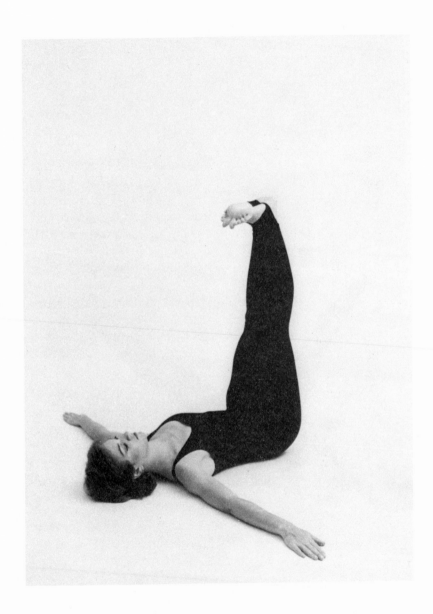

Step 1. Raise both legs together to 90 degrees; hold.

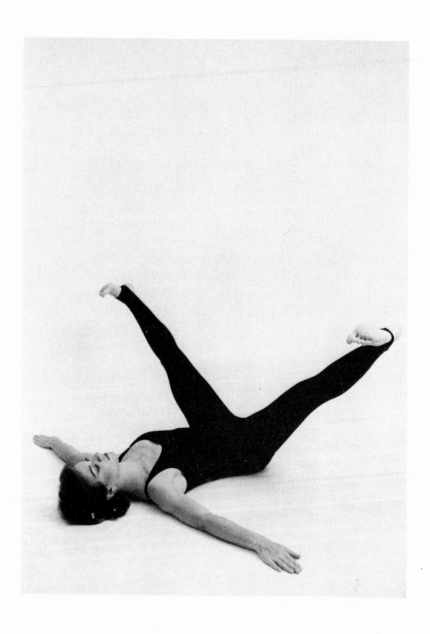

Step 2.   Move legs apart and together again.

Right-Angle-Split Circles from a Supine Position

Lie down on your back to start.

Move arms straight out to the sides (cross position).

Palms should be kept flat down.

Press lower back down (lumbar flattening technique).

1. Raise both legs together with locked knees straight up to a right angle or as close to 90 degrees as possible, while still keeping lower back flat on the ground, and *hold*; then split both legs as far apart as possible and *hold*. Next, with legs wide apart, make circles, bringing them together and apart, using an outward leg rotation with flexed feet.
2. Try to keep both legs straight and the lower back flat.
3. Keep head down and relaxed—keep chin away from your throat.
4. Keep torso, back straight; do not twist body.
5. The distance apart of your split circles will be determined by your hip and leg flexibility, so be careful not to split your legs too far apart.

Advanced level: 5 times around, reverse direction

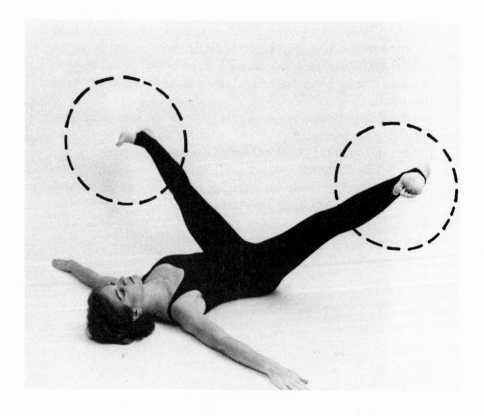

Step 1.   Split legs apart and hold; make circles, bringing legs together and apart.

Saddle Sit-ups from a Right-Angle-Split Position

Lie down on your back to start.

Move arms straight over your head.

Raise both legs together with locked knees straight up to a right angle or as close to 90 degrees as possible, while still keeping your lower back flat on the ground, and *hold*; then split your legs wide apart and *hold*, using a medial leg rotation with flexed feet.

1. Keeping your arms straight and shoulder width apart, *sit up* as far as you can, bringing your arms through your legs.
2. Try to curl your spine as much as possible when sitting up.
3. Keep legs in split position, don't move them when you sit up.

Beginner level: 3–5 reps.

Intermediate level: 5–10 reps.

Advanced level: 5–20 reps.

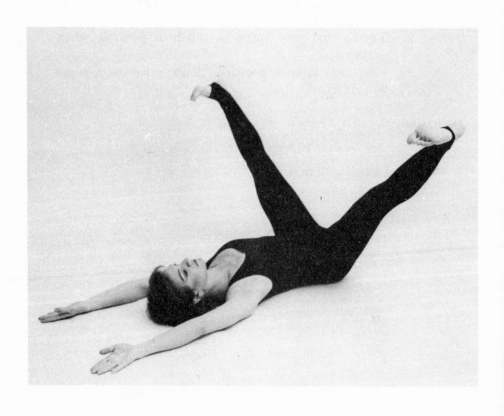

Step 1.   Legs together, up and hold; split and hold.

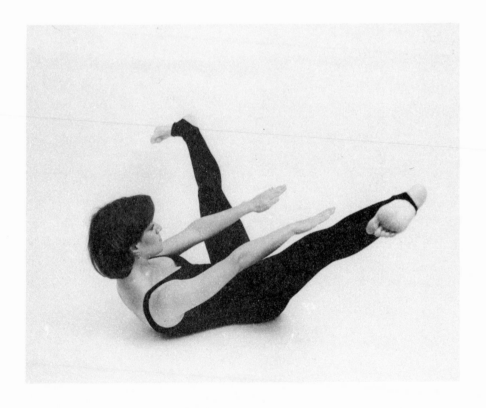

Step 2.   Sit up as far as you can, bringing arms through legs.

Conclusion

CELLULITE IS A FACT of life for those women who don't take good care of themselves. Having cellulite is not a disease or a health problem, but an unesthetic condition that disfigures the body. In a society of automation and overindulgence, exercise and a good diet are needed; furthermore, they are requirements for any woman who wishes to keep her body cellulite-free.

Bibliography

Anderson, W. G. *Best Methods of Teaching Gymnastics*. New York: Hinds, Noble and Eldridge, 1896.

Barlow, W. *The Alexander Technique*. New York: Knopf, 1976.

Chaffee, E. E. and Greisheimer, E. M. *Basic Physiology and Anatomy*. 2nd ed. Philadelphia: Lippincott Co., 1969.

Cooper, K. H. *The New Aerobics*. New York: Bantam Books, 1970.

Cratty, B. J. *Movement Behavior and Motor Learning*. 3rd ed. Philadelphia: Lea & Febiger, 1975.

Daniels, L. and Worthingham, E. *Therapeutic Exercise*. 2nd ed. Philadelphia: W. B. Saunders Co., 1977.

de Vries, H. A. *Physiology of Exercise for Physical Education and Athletics*. 2nd ed. Dubuque, Iowa: William C. Brown Co., 1974.

Drury, B. and Schmid, A. *Introduction to Women's Gymnastics*. New York: Hawthorn Books, 1973.

Edington, D. W. and Edgerton, V. R. *The Biology of Physical Activity*. Boston: Houghton Mifflin Co., 1976.

Feitis, R. *Ida Rolf Talks About Rolfing and Physical Reality*. New York: Harper & Row, 1978.

Feldenkrais, M. *Body & Mature Behavior—A Study of Anxiety, Sex, Gravitation & Learning*. New York: International Universities Press, 1975.

Gray, J. *The Psychology of Fear and Stress*. New York: McGraw-Hill Book Co., 1978.

Gulick, L. *Physical Education by Muscular Exercise*. Philadelphia: P. Blakiston's Son & Co., 1904.

Guyton, A. C. *Basic Human Physiology: Normal Function and Mechanisms of Disease.* 2nd ed. Philadelphia: W. B. Saunders Co., 1977.

Higgins, J. P. *Human Movement—An Integrated Approach.* St. Louis: C. V. Mosby Co., 1977.

Hollinshead, W. H. *Functional Anatomy of the Limbs and Back— A Text for Students of the Locomotor Apparatus.* Fourth Edition. Philadelphia: W. B. Saunders Company, 1976.

Hoppenfeld, S. *Physical Examination of the Spine and Extremities.* New York: Appleton-Century-Crofts/A Publishing Division of Prentice-Hall, Inc., 1976.

Johnson, D. *The Protean Body—A Rolfer's View of Human Flexibility.* New York: Harper Colophon Books, 1977.

Johnson, P. B., Updyke, W. F., Stolberg, D. C., and Schaefer, M. *Physical Education: A Problem Solving Approach to Health and Fitness.* New York: Holt, Rinehart and Winston, 1966.

Kendall, H. O., Kendall, F. P., and Wadsworth, G. E. *Muscles, Testing and Function.* 2nd ed. Baltimore: Williams and Wilkins Co., 1971.

Kendall, H. O., Kendall, F. P., and Boynton, D. A. *Posture and Pain.* Huntington, N. Y.: Robert E. Krieger Publishing Co., 1977.

Klafs, C. E., and Arnheim, D. D. *Modern Principles of Athletic Training.* 4th ed. Saint Louis: C. V. Mosby Co., 1977.

Kounovsky, N. *Six Factors of Physical Fitness.* New York: J. H. Augustin, 1946.

Kurtz, R. and Prestera, H. *The Body Reveals—An Illustrated Guide to the Psychology of the Body.* New York: Harper & Row/Quicksilver Books, 1976.

Lowman, C. L., Colestock, C., and Cooper, H. *Corrective Physical Education for Groups.* New York: A. S. Barnes and Co., 1928.

Null, G., and Null, S. *How to Get Rid of the Poisons In Your Body.* New York: Arco Publishing Company, 1977.

Nutrition Search, Inc. *Nutrition Almanac.* New York: McGraw-Hill Book Co., 1979.

Orback, S. *Fat is a Feminist Issue.* New York: Berkley Medallion Books, 1979.

Posse, N. *The Swedish System of Educational Gymnastics.* Boston: Lee & Shepard, 1890.

Pritikin, N., and McGrady, P. M. *The Pritikin Program for Diet and Exercise.* New York: Grosset and Dunlap, 1979.

Rama, Swami, Ballentine, R., and Hymes, A. *Science of Breath (A Practical Guide)*. Honesdale, Pa.: Himalayan International Institute of Yoga Science & Philosphy, 1979.

Rasch, P. J., and Burke, R. K. *Kinesiology and Applied Anatomy*. 5th ed. Philadelphia: Lea and Fibiher, 1977.

Reich, W. *The Functions of Orgasm*. New York: Pocket Books, 1978.

Roaf, R. *Posture*. New York: Academic Press, 1977.

Rolf, I. P. *Rolfing—The Integration of Human Structure*. Santa Monica, Calif.: Dennis-Landman, 1977.

Ronsard, N. *Cellulite: Those lumps, bumps and bulges you couldn't lose before*. New York: Bantam Books, 1975.

Runner's World Magazine. *Runner's Training Guide*. Mountain View, Calif.: World Publications, 1975.

Selkurt, E. E. *Physiology*. 4th ed. Boston: Little, Brown and Co., 1976.

Selye, H. *The Stress of Life—A New Theory of Disease*. New York: McGraw-Hill, 1976.

Shawn, T. *Every Little Movement—A Book About Francois Delsarte*. 2nd ed. New York: Dance Horizons, 1963.

Siedentop, D. *Physical Education—Introductory Analysis*. Dubuque, Iowa: Wm. C. Brown Co., 1972.

Skarstrom, W. *Gymnastics Kinesiology*. Springfield, Mass.: F. A. Bassette Co., 1909.

Spence, A. P., and Mason, F. B. *Human Anatomy and Physiology*. Menlo Park, Calif.: Benjamin Cummings, 1979.

Sweirgard, L. E. *Human Movement Potential—Its Ideokinetic Facilitation*. 2nd ed. New York: Dodd, Mead & Co., 1975.

Thomas, C. L., ed. *Taber's Cyclopedic Medical Dictionary*. 12th ed. Philadelphia: F. A. Davis Co. 1976.

Thompson, A. *A Handbook of Anatomy for Art Students*. 5th ed. New York: Dover, 1964.

Todd, M. E. *The Thinking Body*. New York: Dance Horizons, 1975.

———*Early Writings 1920-1934*. New York: Dance Horizons, 1977.

Wheeler, R. H., and Hooley, A. M. *Physical Education for the Handicapped*. 2nd ed. Philadelphia: Febiger, 1976.

Zeigler, E. F. *Problems In the History and Philosophy of Physical Education and Sport*. Englewood Cliffs, N. J.: Prentice-Hall, 1968.